Praise for *Introduction to Healthcare Knowledge and Library Services*

'The editors of this compilation have done a marvellous job by bringing together a set of excellent contributions with practical insights from experienced health information professionals in England. They remind us that one is not required to read the book chronologically chapter by chapter, and in fact, I find this to be one of the strengths of the book. While the first chapter sets the background by providing an overview of how NHS England works and what role the library and information services sector plays in this, each of the remaining chapters provides in-depth practitioner-based description and analysis of different aspects of health information services; for example, how these services contribute to the evidence-based practices in healthcare, facilitate the day-to-day activities and decision making of medical professionals, support research, engage in partnership building and advocacy, promote health literacy in the community, and so on. This book covers almost everything that one needs to know about the depth and breadth of the health information services sector, and thus it will serve as an excellent handbook for both present and future health information professionals and researchers in the UK and elsewhere in the world.'
G. G. Chowdhury, Professor of Information Science, University of Strathclyde

'*Introduction to Healthcare Knowledge and Library Services* provides an excellent introduction to the increasingly important area of healthcare knowledge and library services. Each of the 12 chapters, written by leading health information practitioners, provides easy-to-read in-depth looks at a different aspect of healthcare knowledge and library services – ranging from strategic development to training development needs, to evidence-based practice, to the role of partnership and collaboration, to resource discovery and open access, to future opportunities and challenges. The 29 case studies are especially valuable as they help to bring the content to life by portraying actual real-world examples. While the book's chapters specifically focus on the context of the NHS, much of the book provides foundational content that could be applicable to the healthcare knowledge and library services environments in other countries as well. With the growing complexity of the health industry and increasing need to develop health literacy skills to combat misinformation, this book is a timely contribution and a must-read for those interested in working in the healthcare knowledge and library services space and for those who are currently working in the space who may want to expand their knowledge base.'
Dr Sandra Hirsh, Associate Dean for Academics in the College of Professional and Global Education, San José State University, USA

'This book is an exceptional collection of institutional memory of the various shades of library and knowledge development within the NHS. It brings together a wealth of experience from a group of experts which is translated into a comprehensive textbook for anyone new to or experienced in healthcare knowledge and library services. New entrants to the profession, or librarians considering a move to health from other sectors will find this an invaluable point of reference. The case studies give a glimpse into the diversity and range of practice in the field. This book shines a light on the value library and knowledge workers bring to health services and the continued opportunity for advancing healthcare for the next generation. This is an inspiring read and I am so glad the editors managed to capture some of the vast knowledge of the expert contributors, some of whom have since retired. This is a must-read for anyone working in health library and knowledge services.'

Aoife Lawton, National Health Service Librarian, Health Service Executive, Ireland

Introduction to Healthcare Knowledge and Library Services

Introduction to Healthcare Knowledge and Library Services

Edited by
Geoff Walton, Frances Johnson,
David Stewart, Gil Young and
Holly Case Wyatt

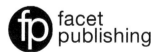

facet
publishing

Published by Facet Publishing
c/o British Library, 96 Euston Road, London NW1 2DB
www.facetpublishing.co.uk

Facet Publishing is wholly owned by CILIP: the Library and Information Association.

British Library Cataloguing in Publication Data
A catalogue record for this book is available from the British Library.

ISBN 978-1-78330-593-3 (paperback)
ISBN 978-1-78330-594-0 (hardback)
ISBN 978-1-78330-595-7 (PDF)
ISBN 978-1-78330-596-4 (EPUB)

First published 2024

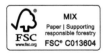

Typeset from editors' files in 10.5/13 Revival 565 and Frutiger by Flagholme Publishing Services.
Printed and made in Great Britain by CPI Group (UK) Ltd, Croydon, CR0 4YY.

Contents

viii   INTRODUCTION TO HEALTHCARE KNOWLEDGE AND LIBRARY SERVICES

Figures, Tables and Case Studies

Figures

Tables

Case Studies

Notes on Contributors

Editors
Holly Case Wyatt has worked in libraries for 12 years, starting in public libraries specialising in health and wellbeing. In 2013, the project *Domestic Abuse, How Surrey Libraries Can Help*, led by Holly, won CILIP's Libraries Change Lives Award. Since joining the NHS in 2015, Holly has worked as an Outreach Librarian delivering library services to NHS staff working in the community and as a Knowledge and Library Development Manager at Health Education England, providing professional advisory guidance and quality assurance of knowledge services to NHS organisations. Holly has a master's degree in Library and Information Management and is a Chartered Member of CILIP. Holly is currently Head of Library Services and Knowledge Management, Surrey and Sussex Healthcare NHS Trust, having previously been the NHS Liaison and Evidence Services Manager at Imperial College London.

Frances Johnson is a Senior Lecturer in the Department of Information and Communications at Manchester Metropolitan University. She has a PhD in Computer Science/Natural Language Processing from the University of Manchester and her field of expertise is in search technologies, information seeking behaviour and user experience (UX). She is currently Associate Editor for *Data Technologies and Applications* and Features Editor for the *Health Information and Libraries Journal*.

David Stewart was Head of NHS Knowledge and Library Services North for Health Education England until his retirement in March 2021. Appointed in 1999, David was responsible for leading the strategic development, co-ordination and monitoring of all NHS knowledge and library services across the North of England. Previous posts include Director of Information Services at the Royal Society of Medicine; Deputy Director of Health Libraries in Oxford Region; and District Librarian for Medway Health Authority. David was CILIP Vice President in 2018 and President in 2019 and served as a CILIP Trustee between 2015 and 2017. He has also chaired CILIP's Health Libraries Group and the NHS Regional Librarians Group. He was the founder of the CHILL network in London and the co-founder of the HEALER network, which brought together a wide range of people interested in health libraries research. Always in demand as a speaker, David has contributed to the professional literature at conferences and through publication in CILIP's *Information Professional* magazine and *Health Information Libraries Journal*. David obtained his CILIP Fellowship in 2012 and was awarded an MBE in the New Year's Honours in 2021.

Geoff Walton is Reader in Information and Digital Literacies in the iSchool at Manchester Metropolitan University. He is currently working on the AHRC-funded project 'Untold Stories: 75th Anniversary of the NHS'. He has recently completed four funded projects: two for the CILIP Information Literacy Group and two ERDF-funded projects (to create an e-learning portal for Jeff Gosling Hand-Controls, the leading UK manufacturer of adaptive engineering for cars, and a User Experience project for the Insights People). His main research interests are information literacy, information behaviour, technology enhanced learning, data literacy and public libraries.

Gil Young has worked in the academic, health and public library sectors. She is currently employed as a Knowledge and Library Services Development Manager, NHS England as part of a national team providing strategic leadership and vision to enable all NHS staff and learners to benefit equally from high quality knowledge and library services. She is a CILIP Fellow and an associate member of the CIPD. Gil is a CILIP Professional Support Officer and was the first winner of the CILIP Mentor of the Year award. She is co-author of *Practical Tips for Developing Your Staff*, published by Facet Publishing.

Contributors

Alison Brettle is a Professor of Health Information and Evidence-Based Practice at the University of Salford. She trained as an information specialist and worked as part of research teams on a range of evidence-based practice related projects in health and social care before developing her own career as an academic. Alison has undertaken systematic reviews relating to library practice and conducted research evaluating the impact of health library services. More recently, she has undertaken research using digital applications and social media to provide information to improve the health of patients with long-term conditions and pregnant women. She actively promotes library practitioner research through her work with the Library and Information Research Group and the International Evidence Based Library and Information Practice movement.

Ruth Carlyle works for NHS England as Head of NHS Knowledge and Library Services. She trained as an information scientist in the pharmaceutical sector before taking health librarian roles in the voluntary sector, notably at the Motor Neurone Disease Association, the Multiple Sclerosis Society and Macmillan Cancer Support. Ruth moved into her role at Health Education England (now NHS England) in April 2017. Her doctorate is on the politics of public involvement in decision-making in the NHS.

Rachel Cooke has been Deputy Director of People and Culture at Surrey and Sussex Healthcare NHS Trust since February 2023, with responsibility for education, learning and development, organisational development and library and knowledge services. Prior to that, Rachel was Head of Library Services and Knowledge Management for Surrey and Sussex Healthcare from 2002 to 2023 (including over three years on secondment, firstly to the NHS Institute for Innovation and Improvement and then to NHS East of England). She has worked in the NHS for over 35 years, in three frontline library service posts, two regional posts (for a total of 14 years) and a secondment as Knowledge Management Fellow to the NHS Institute for Innovation and Improvement, where she also completed the USA-based IHI Quality Improvement Advisor Programme. Building on her interest in QI, Rachel has completed the Lean for Leaders programme and Advanced Lean training.

Alison Day has worked in healthcare libraries for over 18 years and has led on the development of knowledge and library strategies for four NHS foundation trusts and contributed to the development of the national strategy for NHS knowledge and library services, Knowledge for Healthcare. Alison now works in the national Knowledge and Library Services team at NHS England, providing professional advisory guidance and quality assurance of knowledge services to NHS organisations and implementing the national strategy. Alison has a master's degree in Information and Library Studies and is one of the first people to become a CILIP Knowledge Management Fellow.

Clare Edwards has worked in knowledge and library services in the NHS since 1995, working in a variety of roles, including Assistant Librarian and Knowledge and Library Manager, and in regional workforce development, programme co-ordination and strategic roles. In Clare's current role as Deputy Head of Knowledge and Library Services in the NHS England national Knowledge and Library Services team, she works with regional knowledge and library service networks and is the national Knowledge for Healthcare workstream lead for quality, improvement and impact.

Dominic Gilroy has worked in health libraries within the NHS for over 20 years. During that time, he has undertaken a variety of roles, including Information Skills Trainer and Site Librarian, and has managed knowledge and library services in both Acute and Mental Health NHS Trusts. He holds a Fellowship in CILIP and is a Leading Practitioner within the Federation for Informatics Professionals (FEDIP). In his current role as Workforce Planning and Development Lead for the Knowledge for Healthcare workstream within NHS England, he is responsible for managing a range of activities to support the current and future healthcare knowledge and library workforce.

Hélène Gorring has worked in healthcare for over 20 years. Early in her career, she developed an Open Learning Centre for Birmingham Social Services and was then Library Manager at Coventry Primary Care NHS Trust and Birmingham and Solihull Mental Health NHS Trust. She currently works in the Knowledge and Library Services team at NHS England. Hélène was a member of CILIP's Health Libraries Group for many years, where she revamped the Core Collections series of books and, as International Officer, worked with the charity Partnerships in Health Information.

Louise Goswami has worked in regional and national knowledge and library service roles in the NHS for over 18 years. She currently works for NHS England as Deputy Chief Knowledge Officer. Louise played a significant role in the development of the national strategy for NHS Knowledge and Library Services, Knowledge for Healthcare, and was the initial Programme Lead for the implementation of this work. Before joining the NHS, Louise worked as a Knowledge Manager for Accenture and Information Scientist for Hewlett Packard. She has master's degrees in Library and Information Management, Business Administration and Healthcare Leadership. Louise is a Chartered Member of CILIP.

Dawn Grundy is Knowledge and Library Service Lead at Bolton NHS Foundation Trust. Prior to moving to the NHS, she worked in academic libraries supporting healthcare students and academics for over 20 years. Dawn was part of a project team that won the LILAC Digital Literacy Award in 2018, achieved Senior Fellowship of the Higher Education Academy (SFHEA) in 2021 and was awarded CILIP Fellowship in 2023. Dawn co-leads a Health Partnerships Community of Practice and is the national lead for Health Information Week.

Emily Hopkins is Knowledge Management Service Lead at NHS England Workforce, Training and Education Directorate, and is a Chartered

Knowledge Management Fellow of CILIP, a FEDIP Leading Practitioner and a graduate of the University of Sheffield. Emily has developed and delivered knowledge and information services in various settings within the health sector. She has an interest in improving evidence-based decision-making and knowledge mobilisation, including through the development of taxonomies to share organisational knowledge and data, and improving the user experience of search.

Emily Hurt has over 20 years' experience of working in libraries. She has held a variety of roles in three different library sectors: public, higher education and health. In 2018, she won the LILAC Information Literacy Award, awarded to outstanding researchers or practitioners in information literacy.

Sue Lacey Bryant is Chief Knowledge Officer, NHS England. The role encompasses responsibility as the national Lead for NHS Knowledge and Library Services and also as national Head of Profession. Sue has extensive experience of developing knowledge services and managing change in the NHS. She has worked in the private sector and independently as well as enjoying a long career in the NHS in England. Formerly Director of a Clinical Commissioning Group, she is passionate about knowledge management and quality improvement. Taking a leading role in the ground-breaking Topol Review, she then initiated the CILIP Technology Review. She is an Executive Coach. Sue is widely published and was the recipient of the Walford Award in 2018. Currently, Sue is Chair of the CILIP board of trustees.

Siobhan Linsey is the Knowledge and Library Service Manager at Lancashire Teaching Hospitals. Her 20-year career spans primary and secondary education, media research, the book trade and school and health libraries. Trained in coaching and passionate about service development, Siobhan is committed to developing and enabling others and advocates for properly understanding user needs to re-imagine the scope of health library services.

Catherine McLaren has worked in NHS libraries for almost 20 years. During this time, she has undertaken a number of roles including Knowledge Management Lead, Clinical Librarian and as Library Manager in an Acute NHS Trust. She has worked in both regional and national roles. She is a Chartered Member of CILIP and is the Co-Chair for the CILIP Disability Network. She is currently Principal Lead – Knowledge Management & Discovery for NHS Education for Scotland and previously focused on the delivery of Knowledge for Healthcare in NHS England, especially the

Workforce Planning and Development and Health Literacy and Patient Information workstream.

Joanne Naughton joined the NHS in 2001 and worked as a Library and Knowledge Services Manager for 16 years in the acute sector through a period of rapid change in the NHS. Since 2016, she has worked in Health Education England and then NHS England as an NHS Knowledge and Library Services Development Manager. Her role involves regional advocacy, supporting professional development and quality assurance in NHS knowledge and library services. She also works as part of a national Health Literacy and Patient Information team to raise awareness and deliver training on health and digital literacy.

Katie Nicholas is a Knowledge Specialist in the Knowledge Management Service, NHS England Workforce, Training and Education Directorate. Katie has worked in NHS libraries for almost ten years and has been in her current post as a Knowledge Specialist since December 2015, completing a master's in Library and Information Management in the Summer of 2017. Katie helps staff keep up to date with the latest research, supports them in using the evidence base by providing literature searches and summaries, and connects people to people in the organisation through organising and facilitating knowledge sharing events.

Tracey Pratchett is a library and knowledge professional with over 20 years' experience working in health information, further education and public libraries. Now at Citizens' Advice Bureau, she has 16 years' experience working in the healthcare sector, including a knowledge management position at NHS England, facilitating the use of evidence, insights and learning to underpin policy. A qualified teacher and coach, she has extensive experience of encouraging students, healthcare professionals and library and knowledge professionals to use reflective practice to develop themselves and progress their careers.

Victoria Treadway has worked in NHS knowledge and library services since 2004 in a wide range of roles, including Clinical Librarian, Library Services Manager and Knowledge Manager. Victoria works alongside healthcare professionals and teams to understand their knowledge requirements and deliver accessible and responsive services. She is currently a Senior Knowledge Manager at NHS England. Victoria volunteers on the CILIP North West member network as a Professional Registration Support Officer, supporting candidates to achieve CILIP professional registration.

Fran Wilkie started her working life in the library at the University of Salford. After gaining her library and information management qualification, she moved into the NHS where she's now worked for more than 20 years. Her first NHS job was as a library and knowledge skills trainer. Since then, she's held a variety of roles in national organisations providing resources for the NHS, such as the National Library for Health and NICE. She currently works in the Knowledge and Library Services team at NHS England.

Foreword

Rob Webster CBE, Chief Executive,
NHS West Yorkshire Integrated Care Board

The world moves on. Change is a constant. So, how do you discern the truth in our ever-changing world?

Health systems across the globe face many similar challenges: ageing populations, often with multiple health conditions; pressure on resources, both financial and human; harnessing emerging technologies to improve healthcare; the impact of climate change and conflicts; finding the best ways to work in partnership; and ensuring that healthcare is managed and delivered in ways that are truly designed for local populations and are fair and inclusive for everyone in society.

In my part of Yorkshire, I lead a new organisation, an Integrated Care Board, where all these issues are part of the 'everyday' in providing health and social care to 2.4 million people. Working together, all the NHS organisations in West Yorkshire, including primary care as well as local councils and voluntary organisations, are committed to:

- Improving health outcomes for all people using information, data and insight
- Tackling inequality in experiences, outcomes and access
- Enhancing value for money and productivity
- Helping support broader social and economic development.

We understand that information, data and insight are crucial in delivering our plans. Knowledge and library specialists are part of the highly skilled workforce that help us ensure that everything we do, from executive decision-making to frontline care, from treating complex conditions in big teaching hospitals to everyday care in general practice, is informed by evidence from research and by the experience and the know-how of our staff.

In 2021, writing in support of England's national strategy for the development of knowledge and library services, Knowledge for Healthcare, I said, 'Our library and knowledge service enables us to be a learning organisation, ensuring our staff are well supported to make informed decisions and drive innovation.'

Two years on, that is truer than ever. Knowledge and library staff must be an indispensable part of a healthcare system that is changing rapidly and needs fast, reliable and trustworthy information to enable healthcare staff to feel confident that every intervention and clinical decision is underpinned by evidence and best practice.

Making sure we have a well trained health knowledge and library workforce is as important as making sure we have well trained doctors and nurses. So, I am delighted to see this book published as an introduction to the world of health knowledge management and librarianship. I sincerely hope it encourages people around the world to join the profession. For all its challenges, healthcare is an exciting, stimulating and, more than anything, a rewarding world. Please join us.

I was once told, 'if you want to know the truth, ask a librarian'. When change is a constant and the world moves on, this remains sound advice. In this ever-changing world, knowledge and library specialists can help – and they stand ready to make a difference.

How to Use this Book

Geoff Walton and Frances Johnson

This book brings together health information practitioners with a huge variety of experience across health information work within healthcare knowledge and library services in the NHS in England. If there is one overarching message that can be taken away from this book, it is that healthcare knowledge and library services offer a valuable gift to their medical practitioner colleagues – the 'gift of time'. This clearly shows why these services offer vital ongoing support in this important sector.

Each chapter focuses on an essential aspect of health information work and provides a practice handbook and an insight into how health information services operate. The provision of healthcare knowledge and library services continues to develop. With this in mind, it should be noted that Health Education England (HEE), which is mentioned in every chapter, ceased to exist and was replaced by NHS England on 1 April 2023. Given that the vast majority of the work took place under the auspices of the HEE, we felt it fitting to recognise and record that contribution here. The work remains as valuable as ever, but remember to bear in mind that the organisation now has a different name.

The chapters do not need to be read in order and you don't need to read them all. They are standalone, but they are cross-referenced where appropriate. There is a wealth of case studies to show how the ideas put forward here are put into practice. Each chapter has a reference list and there are suggestions for further reading as appropriate.

The book contains an introductory chapter setting the scene and detailing the structure of the NHS and the health information landscape. What follows is a series of in-depth, practitioner focused chapters that describe all aspects of healthcare, knowledge and library work in the health sector.

Chapter 1 is an exploration of the wider healthcare environment, including an overview of the complex structure of the NHS and how the healthcare, knowledge and library services work within this framework.

Chapter 2 foregrounds how the training development needs of health information practitioners are identified and met.

Chapter 3 explains how information, knowledge and library services support the critical area of evidenced-based practice that is necessary for a successful health service.

Chapter 4 describes how information practitioners successfully advocate for their services by building meaningful relationships between the service, medics and decision makers.

Chapter 5 gives an insight into how knowledge is managed within the NHS to maximise its use and benefit to medics.

Chapter 6 closely examines partnerships and collaborative working between the NHS library knowledge services and stakeholders to show how meaningful relationships can be created.

Chapter 7 investigates the developing area of health literacy that is becoming ever more critical in countering and resisting the spread of health misinformation in an era characterised by the so called 'infodemic'.

Chapter 8 gives a detailed account of resource discovery for the NHS in England, including a brief overview of open access publishing and its implication for the sector.

Chapter 9 provides a foundation for doing research to enable readers to carry out robust research that will contribute to the evidence base.

Chapter 10 demonstrates how growing the evidence base of health library and knowledge services contributes to articulating their impact and value.

Chapter 11 provides guidance on how to become a reflective practitioner in the field of health information, knowledge and library work and recognises the value this essential competency brings.

Finally, Chapter 12 looks to the future and what that might bring in terms of opportunities as well as challenges in digital technology and artificial intelligence.

We would like to take this opportunity to thank all of the authors for their time, energy and expertise in creating this new book. We believe it will become an essential handbook for those working in health information and those who are interested in it as students, fellow information practitioners or researchers.

1

An Introduction to Healthcare Knowledge and Library Services

David Stewart and Gil Young

Introduction

Working in a health organisation can be a bewildering experience for new knowledge and library service (KLS) staff. Such organisations often have thousands of highly pressured clinical and managerial staff spread across multiple sites, with little time to explain how things work and what all the jargon means.

The good news is that, as a knowledge and library professional, you are already equipped to do lots of finding out for yourself:

- Start digging, start a set of notes, start a glossary or a set of questions.
- If it helps, draw up organisational and staff structures. A visual representation works better for some people.
- Network with knowledge and library colleagues in other health care organisations.

Our experience shows that these come in useful when you, in turn, are helping new staff understand the complex world they have just joined. One of the authors of this chapter used their diagram of the English National Health Service (NHS) as part of the induction for a finance director who had come from a non-health background, earning his gratitude and a friendly smile ever after.

This chapter will help you structure your voyage of discovery as you work out what your new organisation is all about and how it fits into the wider healthcare system of your country. It will also get you thinking about health in its wider societal context.

As we write, the COVID pandemic is an example of a worldwide issue, affecting every person in every country. Knowledge and library specialists play an important role in enabling fellow health staff, the public, patients, families and carers locate and, crucially, use high quality knowledge resources. The services provided by healthcare knowledge and library services 'take the "heavy lifting" out of getting evidence into practice and give the "gift of time" to healthcare professionals' (Economics by Design, 2020).

A word on terminology before we get started. We will generally use knowledge and library specialist to mean a person qualified in librarianship to at least degree level, or someone who aspires to be. This term covers a broad spectrum of roles across healthcare including, but not limited to, librarian, information professional and knowledge specialist. Most of our examples will come from the NHS but we believe you will be able to take the questions we think you should ask, find the answers and then apply them in your own home setting.

Thinking about numbers and scale

In this chapter, we will be posing several questions and using the NHS as a case study. This should help you think about your knowledge and library service not just in the context of your organisation but also the wider provision of healthcare in your country. If you are not currently employed in this sector, think about a service that is near to where you live or one where you might like to work.

How many staff work in the NHS in England?

There are about 1.2 million full-time equivalent staff (sometimes written as 'FTE' or as 'WTE' for whole time equivalent) working in the NHS in England (NHS Digital, 2022). This will equate to a lot more people as many staff work part-time. When you are looking at this data, check whether you are looking at 'head count' or FTE.

Of these 1.2 million, how many are doctors and nurses?

There are about 118,000 doctors and around 320,000 nurses and midwives across the NHS in England (NHS Digital, 2022). You can see these make up only a fraction of the workforce, yet many people think 'doctors and nurses' when they think about healthcare staff. Often overlooked are other groups such as physiotherapists, occupational therapists and, of course, all those working as administrators, researchers, managers and in other non-clinical roles. Do you know what the breakdown is for all these groups in your organisation? Think about 'managers' as this term will hide a host of other groups of staff: executives, human resources, supplies, finance and IT staff. How is your knowledge and library service supporting their information needs?

What is the significance of '36 hours' to the NHS?

In 2013, it was calculated that the NHS in England sees 1 million patients every 36 hours (The King's Fund, 2023). Even before the COVID pandemic, putting many services under considerable pressure and extending waiting lists. Health Education England, in partnership with The Chartered Institute of Library and Information Professionals (CILIP), launched the #AMillionDecisions campaign (Health Education England, 2021a) to promote the fact that all these treatment interventions need to be evidence based and that as knowledge and library staff you have a key role in providing that evidence. Do you know how many patients are treated each day in your organisation or country?

How many knowledge and library staff are there in the NHS in England?

In April 2021, there were just under 1,008 FTE knowledge and library staff in the NHS in England (Health Education England, 2021b). Again, the headcount is more than this as many staff are employed on a part-time basis. 63% of this small specialist workforce is professionally qualified, the remainder being paraprofessional staff. Other knowledge and library professionals are vitally important for networking, for professional support and development as well as for resource sharing. What do the numbers look like for the organisation or country you are considering? What is the balance between professional and paraprofessional staff and is that balance changing?

Who can make use of NHS knowledge and library services?

Health Education England has NHS-wide responsibility for the strategic development, co-ordination and quality of NHS knowledge and library services in England. Its ambition is that:

> NHS bodies, their staff, learners, patients and the public use the right knowledge and evidence, at the right time, in the right place, enabling high quality decision-making, learning, research and innovation, to achieve excellent healthcare and health improvement.
>
> (Health Education England, 2021c)

NHS knowledge and library services are for all staff and learners, not just for doctors and nurses. Talking to colleagues from other countries, we know that knowledge and library services can be focused on doctors and research and often in academic institutions, but this is not the case in the UK. Who is your knowledge and library service for?

Our Library and Knowledge Service enables us to be a learning organisation, ensuring our staff are well supported to make informed decisions and continue to drive innovation.

(Rob Webster CBE, Chief Executive of South West Yorkshire Partnership NHS Foundation Trust, Lead Chief Executive West Yorkshire and Harrogate Integrated Care System, Health Education England, 2021c)

Moving on to context

There are a wide range of societal factors that affect the provision of healthcare. While these are the important factors in England, many will also apply to other countries, though perhaps with different balances and emphases.

An ageing population

Scientific advances and greater awareness of lifestyle choices mean that many of us are living longer than we would have in the past (Office for National Statistics, 2021a). However, with older age comes a greater risk of disease and infirmity and therefore a growing demand on healthcare and social care systems.

Healthy life expectancy [has] increased over time, but not as much as life expectancy, so more years are spent in poor health …. Similarly, disability-free life expectancy is almost two decades shorter than life expectancy.

(The King's Fund, 2021)

A growing population

In England, there were over 56.5 million people in 2020 (Office for National Statistics, 2021b). It is expected that this will rise to over 59.8 million people by 2040 (Office for National Statistics, 2021c), all needing healthcare throughout their lives. This picture varies around the world, with some countries seeing large projected increases in population through the rest of this century while others are seeing a fall in their predicted populations.

Multiple long-term conditions

As people live longer, so the likelihood that they have more than one health condition increases, putting further pressure on healthcare and social care systems. This includes conditions such as diabetes, hypertension, arthritis and dementia. In England, there are already over 15 million people living with these conditions and this figure is expected to rise as people live longer (The King's Fund, 2013).

Scientific advances

New technologies, drugs and techniques are being made available all the time, making it possible to treat patients more effectively and, sometimes, more quickly. Some of these technologies are expensive to develop, implement and maintain and some need health staff to develop new skills to manage them. As people are better informed than ever before, they know about the latest technologies and treatments and often have expectations that they will be able to access these at their local hospital. Managing public and patient expectations is a challenge for many healthcare systems.

The expert patient

Increasingly, patients are able to learn more about their conditions themselves. They often know more about how they live with, experience and manage their conditions than anyone else, including health professionals. Patients can be recognised as health literate experts in terms of their healthcare. For this reason, they are increasingly being given more choice in terms of treatments, including which treatment pathway they wish to follow and where they want to be treated. There is also an increased emphasis on the importance of patients choosing 'healthy lifestyles', which will avoid them getting sick in the first place and needing healthcare interventions.

Developing the health literacy skills of the healthcare workforce and of patients, families and carers is a growth area for NHS knowledge and library staff in England. What is your role in this field?

The public-private healthcare mix

In England, the NHS is publicly funded and is mostly free at the point of delivery. However, alongside the NHS, there are growing numbers of private health care providers working in partnership with the NHS. Patients may therefore be treated by a private provider 'on the NHS'. You may need to consider what the balance is in your country; there may be a mix of private, public-funded and charitable healthcare providers. How do they work together and which of them have knowledge and library services and staff that you can network with?

Government: legislation and policy

Governments in all countries need to address the challenges and demands outlined above. There will always be 'new plans' for improving healthcare and new policies to implement those plans. Inevitably, health services are subject to politics and in England there have been many reorganisations since the founding of the NHS in 1948. These in turn are likely to affect the overall health system and your organisation, so keep a watching brief on what politicians and thought leaders are saying and what plans they have for the future of healthcare in your country.

Knowledge and library services in more detail

We have used data provided by NHS knowledge and library services in England to provide a more detailed picture of the scale of service provision and the kinds of services offered.

Case Study 1.1: Providing access to high quality information to underpin decisions around healthcare

Team/project lead: Project Knowledge and Library Services / Jane Roberts
Trust: Greater Manchester Mental Health NHS Foundation Trust
Target group: Anyone working within a heath or social care setting in the city of Manchester

The Library and Knowledge Service (LKS) at Greater Manchester Mental Health (GMMH) serves over 5,700 staff across a wide geographical area. GMMH services are based in Bolton, City of Manchester, Salford, Trafford and Wigan. Specialist mental health and substance misuse services are delivered across Greater Manchester and the North West of England.

We have close working relationships with tutors at the Psychological Therapies Training Centre (PTTC) and the Trust's Recovery Academy. The PTTC offers a wide range of cognitive behavioural therapy (CBT) courses to students across England and we work closely with the tutors to ensure students have access to appropriate texts and resources. The Recovery Academy offers mental health and wellbeing courses to staff, students, carers and service users within the Trust and to the public. As part of this offer, the LKS runs shared reading groups and a session on locating high quality health information. Service users at the Trust are provided with study space and computer access at the Curve Library.

The Knowledge Service, based in Fallowfield, forms part of the buzz Health and Wellbeing Service (hereafter buzz). Buzz is commissioned by Manchester Health and Care Commissioning (MHCC), a partnership organisation between Manchester City Council and NHS Manchester Clinical Commissioning Group, delivered by GMMH. Buzz aims to support the health and wellbeing of communities in Manchester and is made up of three teams: Community Development, Physical Activity and Referral Service (PARS) and the Knowledge Service. Our role is to provide anyone working within a healthcare or social care setting in the city of Manchester with access to high quality information to underpin decisions around healthcare. We provide health promotion resources and an evidence search service to buzz and the Manchester Population Health

Team within MHCC. We also deliver our Better Information Programme (BIP). Attendees of the BIP become Knowledge Champions, disseminating key messages from the training throughout healthcare and social care organisations in Manchester.
Key themes: service offer, building relationships, knowledge champions study

Numbers
At the time of writing there are:

- 180 separate NHS knowledge and library services in England (Health Education England, 2021b). These are services with a distinct management structure and budget within an NHS organisation. Some will have more than one service point.
- 498,899 registered users (Health Education England, 2021d) across these 180 services. This figure is made up of directly employed NHS staff as well as students on placement from university programmes, such as medicine, nursing and professions allied to medicine.

The overall funding for these 180 services was over £48.2 million per annum, with 65% of that figure spent on staff costs (Health Education England, 2021d). Specialised staff are key to a good service; a knowledge and library service without staff is just a room full of books, tables and computers. It is the professional knowledge of the library staff that make the difference, adding value, designing, delivering and evaluating the knowledge services provided. However, as we have already seen, staffing numbers are relatively small. The size of knowledge and library teams varies from a solo staff member up to a maximum of 12 FTEs. However, many teams operate with less than five or six staff in total.

The services provided
Some of the services offered by NHS knowledge and library services can be characterised as the long established range of offers that have been part of NHS knowledge and library services for decades:

- Searching, summarising and synthesising evidence is increasingly seen as a core service in NHS England, where knowledge and library staff search efficiently and effectively, saving NHS staff time (Economics by Design, 2020).
- Alerts and current awareness services enable staff to keep up to date in their specialist fields.

- Information skills training is important to support those that want to search for themselves, including students with assignments that require they demonstrate search skills.
- Document supply is increasingly digital for journal articles but there has been less take up of e-books in the NHS. Knowledge and library service users still seem to want to borrow print copies of books.
- Many NHS knowledge and library services have a physical space with areas for quiet individual and group study. Albeit small, these spaces challenge designers to come up with solutions to maximise the space available and make them modern and welcoming. Some NHS organisations simply do not lend themselves to providing a physical space, for example, ambulance or mental health trusts spread over large geographical areas and several hundred buildings. Here, a digital service is more likely to be provided, with services accessible via e-mail, telephone and the internet.

Embedded roles, such as clinical or outreach librarians, are still sometimes seen as 'new' even though the first references to clinical librarians in the UK date from the mid-1970s (Farmer, 1977). Such roles are essential in enabling high quality decision-making across the NHS based upon timely access to the best available evidence (Health Education England, 2021e). Not all NHS knowledge and library services have designated posts such as clinical librarian or outreach librarian; the function of these roles is frequently taken on by an assistant librarian or the service manager, depending on the size and structure of the service.

As the concepts of knowledge management (often referred to as knowledge mobilisation) and health literacy have developed over the last 20 to 30 years, NHS knowledge and library services have incorporated elements of a knowledge management approach into their service offer. Currently, these services are not evenly spread across England and there are clearly pockets of good practice. The services below have developed more recently:

- Managing grey literature: the health sector produces a huge amount of literature not published through traditional means and that can be hard to find. Increasingly, paper copies of older reports are difficult and time-consuming to source. At the same time, digital reports often disappear after a website is superseded or refreshed and the links break. Collections such as the National Grey Literature Collection (https://allcatsrgrey.org.uk/wp) offer a nationally co-ordinated approach to collecting, finding and obtaining this kind of information.

- Involvement in a range of knowledge management activities, such as Lessons Learned and Randomised Coffee Trials: these put people in touch with other people to create networks and spread 'know-how', putting people in touch with evidence.
- Supporting research: outside the larger NHS teaching hospitals, research departments tend to be small and focused on developing practitioner research skills and 'ground up' research. Knowledge and library staff can play a crucial role in supporting this work, from traditional literature searching services through to teaching information management skills, such as searching and reference management, on research skills programmes.
- We have already referred to the developing role of NHS knowledge and library specialists in the health literacy field, providing or advising on information for patients, carers and the public. You can read more about this in Chapter 7.

Where do NHS knowledge and library services fit in their home organisation?

Knowledge and library services are provided in almost all NHS organisations, both directly funded and managed within the organisation or via a service level agreement or contract with a neighbouring organisation. Those organisations range from big teaching hospitals (for example, in London and large cities such as Manchester and Birmingham) to local district general hospitals, through to specialist trusts for mental health, cancer or children. Beyond that, there are community and ambulance trusts.

Knowledge and library services can be sited in different departments within different NHS Trusts. There is no 'right or wrong' organisational home as so much depends on the enthusiasm of the relevant departmental head and the personalities involved.

The knowledge and library service manager is rarely, if ever, managed by someone with a knowledge and library specialist background, which means that their line managers often have a limited understanding of what the service can offer. Knowledge and library service managers therefore need to find mechanisms to explain what they do and how they make a difference to the whole workforce of the organisation. Chapter 10 covers measuring progress, value and impact.

Funding NHS knowledge and library services in England

> Excellent knowledge services require strategic buy-in, collaboration and commitment to maximise investment, nationally, locally and across health systems.
>
> (Health Education England, 2021c)

Funding for NHS knowledge and library services across England is historically complex, however there are currently attempts to put this on a more equitable footing and provide organisations with guidance about how much they should put into their knowledge and library service. This is very much a work in progress as we write.

Digital services

Many NHS knowledge and library services were early adopters of computers and their applications. Initially for online searching of remote databases and then the introduction of automated catalogue and circulation systems, NHS knowledge and library staff have been keen to take advantage of falling prices and increasing processing power. The arrival of the internet in the 1990s enabled knowledge and library services to move into the digital age and the '24x7 web offer' is now as important as the more traditional face-to-face services. Anecdotally, but unsurprisingly, the COVID pandemic has led to many more knowledge and library services offering online services, including virtual training sessions, reference interviews and inductions. It will be interesting to see how this balance shapes in the future.

Networking

Here, 'networks' refers to people networks rather than the digital kind. For decades, health knowledge and library staff have recognised the value of sharing knowledge, learning together and sharing resources through inter-lending and document supply and there is a range of formal and semi-formal networks that bring knowledge and library staff and services together.

Many of these networks operate at a regional level in England, for example, the Library Information Health Network Northwest (LIHHN – www.lksnorth.nhs.uk/lihnn) and the South and West Information Management System (SWIMS – www.swimsnetwork.nhs.uk). Some networks are subject-specific such as the Psychiatric Libraries Cooperative Scheme (www.plcs.nhs.uk).

National leadership in England

Regional leadership for NHS knowledge and library services across England was established as long ago as 1967 with the appointment of Roy Tabor as the first NHS Regional Library Advisor (Stewart, 2021). Responsible for the strategic co-ordination, development and quality of knowledge and library services across their region, regional librarians were appointed to all NHS regions by the early 2000s.

Over the last five years, a national team with around 25 staff has developed, led by the Chief Knowledge Officer. Part of their work is to lead the development of NHS knowledge and library services across England, providing professional advice and leadership both to employers and to knowledge and library service teams. This sits alongside national work streams that implement the following main components of the current Knowledge for Healthcare Strategy (Health Education England, 2021c):

- Workforce planning and development (see Chapter 3)
- Mobilising knowledge and evidence (see Chapter 5)
- Health literacy (see Chapter 7)
- Resource discovery (see Chapter 8)
- Quality and impact (see Chapter 10).

Each work stream is led by a member of the national team with the support of small working and reference groups to ensure the programme of work is grounded in practice.

Conclusion

As information 'increasingly become[s] the currency of healthcare in the future … our ability to access, understand and interpret it at individual and population level will be a key determinant in the future success of our healthcare system' (Health Education England, 2017). Skilled knowledge and library staff are critical to the business of healthcare. As outlined above, the task that faces knowledge and library staff is a challenging one. They are small in number, but the ambition is that the important and specialised work they do impacts every part of the healthcare system. Health systems and the care they deliver change and adapt all the time and so too must knowledge and library specialists to ensure their teams and services are flexible, fit for purpose and ready to make a difference.

> The services provided [by knowledge and library staff] take the 'heavy lifting' out of getting evidence into practice and give the 'gift of time' to healthcare professionals. Informed decisions improve outcomes, quality of care, patient experience, resource utilisation and operational efficiencies. This is best achieved when healthcare professionals are supported by the right knowledge services, with the right resources and with the right teams and roles.
>
> (Economics by Design, 2020)

References

Economics by Design (2020) *NHS Funded Library and Knowledge Services in England – Value Proposition: The Gift of Time.* www.hee.nhs.uk/our-work/library-knowledge-services/value-proposition-gift-time.

Farmer, J. (1977) Full Members of the Team: Medical Librarians in the Patient Care Setting, *Library Association Record*, **79**, 81–5.

Health Education England (2017) *Framework 15. Health Education England Strategic Framework 2014–2029.* www.hee.nhs.uk/sites/default/files/documents/HEE%20strategic%20framework%202017_1.pdf.

Health Education England (2021a) *Marketing and Campaigns: #AMillionDecisions.* https://library.hee.nhs.uk/about/marketing-and-campaigns.

Health Education England (2021b) *KLS Statistical Return for NHS KLS Staffing in England 2021–22*, unpublished.

Health Education England (2021c) *Knowledge for Healthcare: Mobilising Evidence; Sharing Knowledge; Improving Outcomes. A Strategic Framework for NHS Knowledge and Library Services 2021–2026.* www.hee.nhs.uk/sites/default/files/documents/HEE%20Knowledge%20for%20Healthcare%202021-26%20FINAL.pdf.

Health Education England (2021d) *KLS Statistical Return for NHS KLS Activity in England 2020–21*, unpublished.

Health Education England (2021e) *Clinical Librarian / Embedded Librarian / Knowledge Specialist / Evidence Specialist.* https://library.nhs.uk/employers-leaders/resources-for-role-redesign/clinical-librarian-embedded-librarian-knowledge-specialist-evidence-specialist.

NHS Digital (2022) *NHS Workforce Statistics – October 2021 (Including Selected Provisional Statistics for November 2021).* https://digital.nhs.uk/data-and-information/publications/statistical/nhs-workforce-statistics/october-2021.

Office for National Statistics (2021a) *National Life Tables – Life Expectancy in the UK: 2018 to 2020.* www.ons.gov.uk/peoplepopulationandcommunity/birthsdeathsandmarriages/lifeexpectancies/bulletins/nationallifetablesunitedkingdom/2018to2020.

Office for National Statistics (2021b) *Population Estimates for the UK, England and Wales, Scotland and Northern Ireland: Mid-2020.* www.ons.gov.uk/peoplepopulationandcommunity/populationandmigration/populationestimates/bulletins/annualmidyearpopulationestimates/mid2020#population-change-for-uk-countries.

Office for National Statistics (2021c) *National Population Projections: 2020-Based Interim.* www.ons.gov.uk/peoplepopulationandcommunity/populationandmigration/populationprojections/bulletins/nationalpopulationprojections/2020basedinterim.

Stewart, D. (2021) Roy Tabor 1929–2021: The First NHS Regional Librarian in England, *Health Information and Libraries Journal*, **38** (3), 242–3.

The King's Fund (2013) *Long-Term Conditions and Multi-Morbidity.* www.kingsfund.org.uk/projects/time-think-differently/trends-disease-and-disability-long-term-conditions-multi-morbidity.

The King's Fund (2021) *What is Happening to Life Expectancy in England?* www.kingsfund.org.uk/publications/whats-happening-life-expectancy-england.

The King's Fund (2023) *Activity in the NHS.* www.kingsfund.org.uk/projects/nhs-in-a-nutshell/NHS-activity.

2

Strategic Development for Healthcare Knowledge and Library Services

Louise Goswami, Alison Day and Holly Case Wyatt

Introduction

This chapter examines the importance of having a documented strategy for healthcare knowledge and library services. It discusses how to recognise key drivers for the use of knowledge, information and evidence within the health service and how to use these to inform a strategy, with consideration given to aligning the strategy to both organisational and national priorities. The chapter also explains the need to place stakeholders at the heart of strategic development and describes the seven steps involved in creating a strategy, including evaluating the impact and effectiveness of the healthcare knowledge and library service strategy.

Why is strategy important?

A strategy is intrinsic to delivering an effective healthcare knowledge and library service. It showcases how to support the delivery of organisational priorities, aligning to those priorities and ensuring growth. A strategy demonstrates how a service contributes to the overall success of an organisation, the plan to evolve in the future and outlines where a service makes a positive difference. A well written and thought-out strategy gives structure to important conversations within an organisation, but also with other partners. It will be the foundation of business cases, service change, networking and building relationships with senior stakeholders within an organisation.

To underpin improvement and quality assurance, a well aligned strategy is essential. It can be used to communicate the vision to the team and stakeholders and presents a road map of how to get there. Good strategies should have clear SMART objectives (see Figure 2.1 on the next page) that demonstrate how to use team resources, experience and knowledge to advance the ambitions of an organisation. A key part of developing a strategy is ongoing monitoring and review to measure progress against the targets that have been set.

SMART objectives
Specific or focused, giving details of services and target groups
Measurable, quantifiable
Achievable, within the contexts and resources available
Relevant, in that they contribute to organisational success and are aligned with
   corporate objectives
Timely so that actions are taken at the right time to achieve market success; this
   involves judging market readiness.

Figure 2.1 *SMART objectives* (Roberts and Rowley, 2008, 157)

Hooks and levers

The starting point for any strategic development is to consider what is happening in the world that has an impact on the work the service needs to deliver. This may take a wide view to consider political, economic, sociological, technological, legal and environmental issues, but it will also need to consider national and local health-related concerns. National documents that can drive strategic development include other national strategies, policies and legislation. The health service is awash with national strategic documents and part of the role of strategic development is to demonstrate a causal link between what is written in policy and legislation and demonstrating how it is reflected in the health library service.

For example, in Scotland, recent advice and guidance makes frequent mention of the role of using evidence, stating that 'evidence-based practice sits at the heart of all clinical decision making' (NHS Scotland, 2022). This is an obvious opportunity or hook to demonstrate the need for a healthcare library service to assist with ensuring evidence is used in healthcare practice. Where there is a national knowledge and library services strategy in place, such as Knowledge into Action (NHS Education for Scotland, 2016), interpretation of policy drivers may have already been distilled into additional documents. This is often incorporated into more tailored national knowledge and library service policies or forms part of research, such as the Gift of Time Value Proposition research (Economics by Design, 2020).

You will also need to consider documents produced locally. This will include the strategy and operational plan for all the organisations that receive the library service. It may also require research into the priorities of other stakeholders. These can include the priorities for the local health system or for local education providers where you provide a service to staff, students and learners from those institutions.

Taking time at this stage ensures that the strategy is based on evidence from research and is rooted in the hooks and levers used in the wider healthcare context.

National and local working in tandem

Strategic documents have different functions. The strategy of a local NHS Trust will showcase how the Trust plans to deliver their priorities, drawn down from government drivers and local need. Whereas a document such as Health Education England's Knowledge for Healthcare (Health Education England, 2021) will act as a driver for change. Where a national strategy exists, local services should align their own strategy to that as well as to the strategic priorities of their host organisation. For example, within NHS Knowledge and Library Services in England, a strategy showcases how you will support the delivery of your organisational priorities and those set out in Knowledge for Healthcare, aligning those priorities and ensuring growth.

The business plan example from Barts Health NHS Trust (see Figure 2.2) demonstrates how a service can align priorities to a number of different strategic drivers. The plan starts by reiterating the current vision for the Trust

Barts Health NHS Trust Knowledge and Library Services Business Plan 2021–22						
Trust Vision	To be a high performing group of NHS hospitals, renowned for excellence and compassionate care to our patients in east London and beyond					
Academy	Leading the way in education and learning					
KLS Purpose	Support evidence-based decision-making, clinical governance, clinical effectiveness, research and development, management, education and lifelong learning by **delivering knowledge at the point of need** to all Trust staff and students					
HEE Library Quality Priorities	Proactive KLS meets organisa-tional priorities within K4H framework	Decision-making is underpinned by evidence provided by KLS specialists	KLS specialists proactively support evidence needs of workforce	The right number and skill mix of KLS staff to deliver on organis-ational and K4H priorities	KLS staff improve and innovate based on research and evidence	KLS demon-strates positive impact of the service
Trust Strategic Priorities 2017–23	Safe and Compassion-ate Care	Efficient and Effective Services	Service Transform-ation	Developing Our People	Improving Our Infrastruct-ure	Better Research and Education
Education Academy Priorities 2021–22	**Future Workforce** Provide the future workforce with the right skills to adapt to new ways of delivery	**Current Workforce** Develop current staff in **new technologies** and to support **transform-ation and recovery**	**Quality and Patient Safety** High quality **learning environment** to enhance the patient safety	**Health and Wellbeing** Support emotional health and wellbeing of staff	**Future Workforce** Provide the future workforce with the right skills to adapt to new ways of delivery	

Figure 2.2 *An example of aligning a strategy to meet national and local needs*

KLS Priorities 2021–22	**Current and Future Workforce** To help Trust staff to apply and use evidence, build know-how, continue to learn and drive innovation To ensure the collection is developed to meet the needs of the workforce including staff development of all types, including leadership and management material To provide digital literacy training to ensure staff are able to use the technology available to them To work closely within the Education Academy to support training and development programmes with relevant resource To support Trust staff coming to the library to use computers in order to undertake online training To meet the Equality Agenda by the provision of material for all grades and levels of staff from all backgrounds – to include easy reading, basic numeracy, literacy To provide space for staff to bring their own devices and offer support where needed To provide training in evidence searching and health literacy skills
	Quality and Patient Safety To ensure that staffing, services and resources are aligned to support the evidence and knowledge needs of the Trust To support decision-making at all levels and across the whole Trust, to include clinicians, senior managers, staff at the bedside, admin, purchasing, etc. To work with the WeImprove team to support their evidence and knowledge requirements and plan services to meet Trust developments
	Health and Wellbeing Provide health literacy training to Trust staff, patients, carers and the local population through collaboration with public libraries and other organisations To continue to develop and provide wellbeing resources, including the Wellbeing Evidence Update To ensure the library spaces are suitable spaces for quiet study and reflection

	New Initiatives
	HEE/British Library project to create a shared national NHS repository; Barts Health KLS will lead on the section for Serious Incidents
	Digital Health Champions
	A collaborative project with NELFT, funded by HEE, to enable patients to access virtual clinics by developing their digital skills
	Possibility of HEE funding for merging our current library management system with others in London. This would result in long-term cost savings and possible reduced staff pressure.
	New initiatives from HEE across all NHS libraries which will require staff input at a local level:
	  New e-book platforms
	  New Discovery platform
	  Move to a different search tool
	  Change of link-resolver
	  Digital and Health Literacy delivery requirements

	Mobilising Evidence and Knowledge (HEE) To contribute to the improvement of the knowledge flow across and within the Trust To work collaboratively with other libraries within NE London To support decision-making at all levels and across the whole Trust, to include clinicians, senior managers, staff at the bedside, admin, purchasing, etc.

Figure 2.2 *Continued*

KLS Priorities 2021–22	**Quality and Impact (HEE)** To meet the requirements of the HEE Quality and Improvement Outcomes Framework for NHS Libraries To ensure maximum efficiency and cost effectiveness of services and systems To work collaboratively to allow value for money and efficient working To improve and enhance KLS spaces To develop and improve KLS systems and services						
	Health Literacy and Patient Information (HEE) To support the work and aims of the Patient Experience Committee To contribute to the work of the Patient Information Reference Group To provide health literacy training to Trust staff, patients, carers and the local population through collaboration with public libraries and other organisations To work with local partners (e.g. public libraries) to ensure patients and carers have access to high quality health information To develop a range of resources suitable for supporting and informing patients and carers						
	Quick and Easy Access to Digital Knowledge Resources (HEE) To continue to build on the digital by default strategy, making resources available 'anytime, anywhere' whenever possible To improve access and usage of resources and services To move to personalised services through software options To offer remote training via webinars and podcasts, etc. To support the improvement of the digital literacy of staff, students and patients To align with Trust paperless policy To develop the collection to support learning in new technology/digital subjects, including the creation of alerts and updates for staff						
	Developing the Right Knowledge Services Workforce (HEE) To encourage and support KLS staff to develop the skills and capability to deliver the services required and offer opportunities to become professional practitioners						
Trust	Welcom-ing	Engag-ing	Collaborative	Accountable	Respectful	Equitable	Welcoming
KLS Values	• A high quality customer focused service • Accessible and inclusive • Courteous and friendly • Dynamic and innovative • Professional and accountable						

Figure 2.2 *Continued*

and also reflects the vision statement for the Academy in which the knowledge and library service sits. Next comes the purpose statement for the knowledge and library service. This describes in a nutshell what the service does. A really effective purpose statement, sometimes referred to as a 'mission statement', will utilise key words or phrases from the organisation vision or purpose statement as this helps show alignment with what the overarching organisation is there to achieve.

The example has chosen to include three sets of priorities that guide the work of the service – national Health Education England quality priorities, Trust strategic priorities and the Education Academy priorities. Headings from these overarching priorities are then used to cluster the operational priorities for the service. This can be helpful when sharing information about the work of the service with the library team and wider stakeholders. It sets out a concise view of how the work of the service helps to meet the priorities of the wider Academy and Trust, as well as showing good alignment with the national driver for change. Finally, this plan includes the Trust values and service values, which help to give a sense of the organisational culture that is in place to underpin the work.

The Barts Health Knowledge and Library Service operational plan follows the format of a 'plan on a page'. This is a strategic document that defines your strategic vision and purpose, whilst aligning the priorities of the library service to those of the organisation (Health Education England, 2022). It can be a helpful way of communicating complex information in a format that is easy to read and present, including for marketing and other advocacy purposes.

Working strategically within a wider healthcare system

Aligning the knowledge and library service strategy to the aims and objectives of the host organisation is crucial, however there is also a need to remain aware of opportunities to work at a wider system level. Healthcare is a fluid sector with regular changes to legislation, policy and structure. For example, in July 2022, new legislation in England saw the development of 42 Integrated Care Boards. These became the statutory strategic decision-making bodies of place-based Integrated Care Systems or Partnerships that bring together all organisations involved in providing care services to a local community. This includes NHS care providers such as acute, community, mental health and primary care services; local authority; public health; social care; and third sector organisations. According to the Health and Care Act 2022, each Integrated Care Board must, in the exercise of its functions, facilitate or otherwise promote research on matters relevant to the health service and the use of evidence obtained from research to inform decision-making. This will be assessed and monitored by NHS England.

As healthcare systems develop, knowledge and library services will be required to work across a wider footprint. This will lead to instances where a strategy will need to be co-created with other knowledge and library service providers to ensure consistent delivery.

Placing stakeholders at the heart of developing a strategy

Involving key stakeholders is imperative to the development of a successful strategy. Stakeholders will have put in place priorities and values for the organisation that will act as the cornerstone of a strategic document. Stakeholders include organisational decision makers, advocates for a service and existing and potential users. It is good to have a diverse range of people to consult on a strategy. Strategy development should also consider the needs of library service users.

You can involve stakeholders at any stage of the development of a strategy but it is particularly helpful at the start, to formally approve the strategy and to advocate throughout.

Case Study 2.1: Development of national strategies for knowledge and library services

Team/project lead: NHS Education for Scotland and Healthcare Improvement Scotland / Annette Thain

Knowledge into Action (K2A) has been the key driver shaping NHS Scotland's Library and Knowledge Services since 2016. It is currently being revised.

How did you get started?

Engagement is underway with key organisations to develop a joint understanding of the aims and why this is essential to shape the future role of knowledge and library services.

In preparation, we have also reviewed the current literature, other strategies and examples of good practice. We have envisioned the future with librarians and stakeholders and identified opportunities that demonstrate the benefits of supporting libraries and knowledge services to organisations. We have found it helpful to present the case from the perspective of senior management and leaders.

Who did you work with?

The current work is led by Public Health Scotland, Healthcare Improvement Scotland, NHS Education for Scotland and the Programme Lead, Knowledge and Decision Support, Digital Health & Care Innovation Centre.

How did you approach your strategic development?

To define the original K2A approach, the librarians delivered a serious of tests of change using improvement methodology and evaluated these using a contributions analysis framework. This resulted in the K2A process cycle and the recognition that the implementation required a network approach. One person was unlikely to be able to support all aspects combining research evidence, people's experience and context to produce knowledge assets that are actionable to get the right information, in the right format to the right people at the right time.

During 2022, the K2A approach is to be updated to provide a cohesive direction of travel for the librarians working in partnership with data analysts and others. This will ensure they can continue to support the needs of the health and social care workforce to get knowledge used in practice, taking into consideration the developments in technology, artificial intelligence and decision support. This will include the provision and promotion of the digital library; evidence search and summary services; decision support; digital information literacy skills; knowledge management tools; shared decision-making; and including health literacy, working with the public and school libraries.

You can find out more about K2A here:

https://learn.nes.nhs.scot/2928

(NHS Education for Scotland, 2012)

Key themes: knowledge into action, strategic development, improvement methodology, stakeholder engagement

The case study highlights important elements to consider when developing a strategy. These can be applied to a national strategy, as in the example, but can also be mirrored by any knowledge and library service developing a strategy. Engagement with stakeholders is at the heart of good strategic development. In this case, there was engagement with key organisations and the strategy itself was co-created with partners involved in the delivery and use of knowledge, information and evidence.

The Knowledge into Action approach presents a clear and cohesive direction for healthcare knowledge services in Scotland and acknowledges the need to work with others (for example, data analysts) and to consider developments in technology, artificial intelligence and decision support. The overarching vision 'to support the needs of the health and social care workforce to get knowledge used in practice' aligns closely with the framework for developing a 'learning health system'.

Learning health systems

Knowledge and library specialists have a key role to play in the development of learning health systems (Foley, 2022). The transformation of data, information and evidence into knowledge that can be applied to healthcare decision-making and healthcare practice leads to a cycle of continuous improvement. This is often described as a learning health system: 'an organisation skilled at creating, acquiring and transferring knowledge, and modifying its behaviour to reflect new knowledge and insights' (Foley, Horowitz and Zahran, 2021). For a learning health system to thrive, there needs to be a clear rationale – this is where having a well communicated strategy fits in. Key to any learning health system is the development of a learning culture. Healthcare library and knowledge services contribute to this learning culture by ensuring rapid access to high quality evidence and by promoting good use of knowledge mobilisation techniques to ensure know-how and learning is captured and shared. This, combined with reviews of healthcare information and data, contribute to informed continuous improvement and ensure that care is delivered in a safe environment.

Steps for creating a strategy

Inform your strategy with research

All well informed strategies start with a consideration of the evidence to support the strategic direction of the service.

A good place to begin is to review national guidance and policies relating specifically to knowledge and library services. A review of broader health service documents should also be included. Familiarity with the strategy and delivery plans of the organisations that will use the library service is essential. Within these, there will be ways to align the work of the library service to the priorities for the organisation.

It may be useful to receive regular horizon scan alerts to keep updated about trends and future developments. It is also helpful to look at examples of good practice and policies from elsewhere in the sector that could be adopted locally. Being a member of a community of practice where good practice is shared and questions can be asked can be a great help when developing library strategy.

Analysis

Once you have conducted initial research, it is useful to analyse the current picture by conducting both a PESTLE and a SWOT analysis (Chartered Institute of Personnel and Development (CIPD), 2021a; 2021b). With a PESTLE analysis, consideration is given to the Political, Economic, Sociological, Technological, Legal and Environmental issues that currently exist, or that are predicted may exist in the future, that will impact upon service delivery. A SWOT analysis encourages consideration of the internal and external Strengths, Weaknesses, Opportunities and Threats. This analysis is best conducted by the whole team. If possible, involve stakeholders to help get a broad and diverse range of views.

Stakeholder engagement

Service users and other stakeholders can be invited to workshops to help develop a strategy. In this way, they can contribute to the analysis and generation of ideas. Stakeholders must be consulted once a draft outline of a strategy has been produced. It is useful to test with them the overall vision and purpose or mission statement and to see how they respond to the suggested priorities or objectives. A useful tip is to present the strategy from the perspective of senior management and leaders – framing it in language that aligns to their priorities and demonstrating the benefits of a knowledge and library service. A driver diagram (see Figure 2.3 below) is a simple way to present the overall strategy when getting feedback from stakeholders.

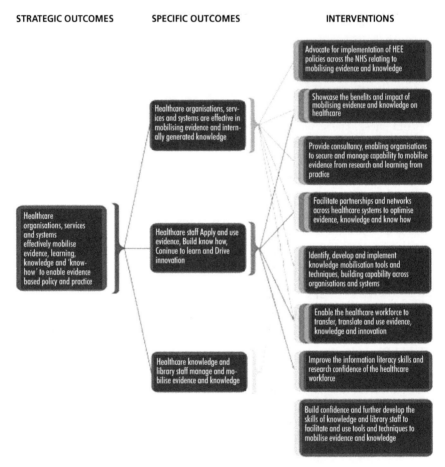

Figure 2.3 *An example of a driver diagram from* Knowledge for Healthcare

Generating ideas – using driver diagrams
Driver diagrams (NHS England and NHS Improvement, 2022) are a useful way to generate and organise a strategy and have been used effectively in the development of both iterations of Knowledge for Healthcare (Health

Education England, 2021). They are simple to use and have multiple benefits: they engage people in the development of a strategy; provide a logical and orderly approach, leading to the avoidance of blind spots; and challenge group-think. There are ten steps to developing driver diagrams:

1 Gather the people with the right expertise together. This could include the knowledge and library services team, key stakeholders and partners.
2 Develop an aim. In the case of Knowledge for Healthcare, this is 'The right evidence and knowledge is used at the right time in the right place'.
3 Identify primary drivers or strategic outcomes. These are a set of factors or areas for improvement that need to be addressed to achieve the desired outcome. These should be written as straightforward statements, not targets.
4 Generate change ideas. Offer as many ideas as possible that might lead to achieving the aim and the primary drivers that have been identified.
5 Look for patterns or themes that seem to be linked.
6 Cluster or 'marshal' the mass of ideas. Linking the ideas provides a new level of secondary drivers or specific outcomes. Each secondary driver will contribute to at least one primary driver. They should be process changes that are expected to impact the outcome and they should have an evidence base. Collectively, they should be necessary and sufficient to achieve the aim.
7 Agree measures. It is important to understand how success will be measured and to develop key performance indicators to help with this.
8 Prioritise. In collaboration with stakeholders and partners, prioritise the work that will be undertaken to deliver the aim.
9 Get started.
10 Share learning.

Advocacy and formal approval

Advocacy and impact are fundamental to strategy development. (Chapter 3 covers in detail the importance of advocacy and impact for healthcare knowledge and library staff.) There is a need to rally stakeholder advocates to ensure that a strategy is formally approved. In addition, stakeholder advocates are needed to ensure the organisation understands how a knowledge and library strategy underpins the priorities of the organisation. This is much easier to achieve if stakeholders are involved from the outset.

The approved strategy can be used as a tool for advocacy to demonstrate the vision and direction of travel for the service and how it contributes to the objectives of the organisation. It forms a central core that drives all service implementation, including development, quality improvement, marketing and resource allocation.

Evaluating the impact of a library strategy

When developing a strategy, it is recommended that time is spent considering how the impact of the strategy will be evaluated, with a focus on achieving outcomes. Outcomes are defined as:

> Changes in behaviour, relationships, activities or actions of people, groups and organisations with whom a programme works directly.
>
> (Earl, Carden and Smutylo, 2001, 1)

A structure for an evaluation framework will need to include impact objectives and indicators and identify the significant processes and activities to ensure progress is being made. Measurement will be through collection of both qualitative evidence and quantitative data in the form of metrics against the impact indicators and processes/activities. Metrics are defined as:

> Criteria against which something is measured.
>
> (Showers, 2015, xxx)

During implementation, there will need to be a process for capturing the measurement of information and data needed to evaluate the strategy. Developing key performance indicators (KPIs) can be a useful way to measure the performance of library and knowledge services, but for maximum effect they need to be linked to quality outcomes such as impact and value (Appleton, 2017). Key performance indicators are defined as:

> … financial and non-financial metrics used to quantify objectives to reflect strategic performance of an organisation.
>
> (SCONUL, 2023)

Implementation and review

Once the knowledge and library strategy has been formally approved by the organisation, an implementation plan can be developed. This will drill down into the operational priorities that need to be put in place and lays out for the team how the strategy will be put into practice. The implementation plan also describes the activities and associated resources that are required to deliver the strategy. This includes who will lead on each aspect of the work; which stakeholders need to be involved; timeframes; risks; and dependencies. This becomes a detailed document to inform the work of the entire team. The strategy and implementation plan will also feed directly into the objectives of the annual development review for each member of the team.

The strategy will inform the approach to marketing and promoting the service by providing a focus on what is strategically important. Strategic marketing has a greater impact within the organisation than more generalised promotion (Kendrick, 2021).

Strategies should be living documents that are regularly reviewed against the work of the service and adapted to address any additional needs that arise. It is also important that they are refreshed or re-written on a regular basis. Although ownership will sit with the manager of the service, all staff should have a working knowledge of the strategy and the part they play in the strategic direction of the service.

Case Study 2.2: Development of the national strategy for the National Health Library and Knowledge Service in Ireland

Team/project lead: Health Service Executive, Health Library Ireland / Aoife Lawton

The Strategy and Implementation Plan for the National Health Library and Knowledge Service in Ireland was commissioned in 2017. The full cycle of work, taking into account the initial tendering process to the eventual publication of the strategy, took nine months. A Strategy Advisory Group was set up with key internal and external stakeholders; two consultation workshops were held in different HSE locations; visits to some library sites were carried out; and an international panel of library and knowledge experts was convened to garner their input and expert opinion during its development.

How did you get started?

I started by securing senior management buy-in and approval to go to tender. A co-design approach was used, which I would recommend as a strong element of the strategy. This approach ensured that all key stakeholders had shared ownership and commitment to the strategy. The inclusion of current and future users of the library and knowledge service, library staff, an international panel of experts and a strategic advisory group was a particularly good approach. It is vital that the strategy aligns with strategic reports and the objectives of the parent organisation at the time.

Who did you work with?

I worked with external consultants who were responsible for the resulting strategy. As one of the consultants, Dr Ann Wales, is already widely recognised as an expert in this field, it was a perfect fit for our service.

What did the resulting strategy look like?
The strategy was launched in March 2018 and is a short nine-page document. This is important because healthcare leaders and managers are time poor, so a short concise strategy was well received.

What is the next stage of development?
2023 is the last year of implementation so plans for a new strategy will be underway. Some elements of the strategy will need revision and testing as implementation takes place. The implementation of the strategy was centred around virtual working and virtual teams. This was accelerated during the pandemic and remains 'how we do business' today.

What is the key message of this strategy?
A core pillar of the strategy was to provide a National Digital Knowledge Gateway, since described as a National eHealth Library. Much has been achieved to deliver this, but there is still some work to do, which is largely funding dependent. The service has since been renamed 'Health Library Ireland' and was launched in September 2022.

You can find out more about Health Library Ireland and access a copy of the latest strategy at https://hselibrary.ie.

(National Health Library and Knowledge Service, 2018)

Key themes: knowledge into action, strategic development, strategic review, stakeholder engagement, co-design, timing

---

Allowing sufficient time to engage with stakeholders is a key message within this case study example from Health Library Ireland. It also demonstrates that developing strategy does not stop with the production of a document. Good strategic development is an ongoing process involving: consulting with stakeholders; acting on feedback; monitoring progress against identified goals or objectives; and modifying the strategy to adjust to changes in wider healthcare policy or to react to other external factors. For Health Library Ireland, this is demonstrated by the way they accelerated the focus on virtual teams and virtual work as a result of the pandemic.

As healthcare systems and organisations evolve, strategies will change and adapt. This must be reflected in the health library service strategy so that it remains aligned to the overall strategic priorities of the organisation.

Waiting for confirmation or sign-off of the organisational priorities with which the library needs to align can often delay the development of the library strategy. This can be the case when an organisation is going through major changes, such as a merger with another organisation. It is more critical that the library service has a strategy to guide and communicate service delivery at these times. Without organisational objectives in place, the service may need to align just to the national drivers for healthcare. This can form an interim or living strategy document that will continue to be adapted as the organisational priorities are confirmed.

Conclusion

A strategy is intrinsic to delivering an effective healthcare knowledge and library service. It will showcase how the knowledge and library service supports the delivery of organisational priorities, aligns to those priorities and ensures growth. It is important to identify the key drivers that will underpin the development of a strategy, including key documents, legislation and policies. Aligning strategy to both national, organisational and departmental priorities helps position the service as business-critical.

Placing stakeholders at the heart of developing a strategy is key. Stakeholders can be involved at any stage but it is particularly helpful at the start, to formally approve the strategy and to advocate throughout. It is also important to spend time considering how the impact of the strategy will be measured.

Strategies should be living documents that are regularly reviewed against the work of the service and adapted to address any additional needs that arise.

Developing a strategy can seem a daunting task. However, by following a step-by-step approach – as outlined in the chapter – it becomes far less intimidating and much more straightforward.

References

Appleton, L. (2017) *Libraries and Key Performance Indicators: A Framework for Practitioners*, Elsevier.

Barts Health NHS Trust (2021) *Knowledge and Library Service Business Plan 2021–2022*, unpublished.

Chartered Institute of Personnel and Development (CIPD) (2021a) *PESTLE Analysis Factsheet*. www.cipd.co.uk/knowledge/strategy/organisational-development/pestle-analysis-factsheet.

Chartered Institute of Personnel and Development (CIPD) (2021b) *SWOT Analysis Factsheet*. www.cipd.co.uk/knowledge/strategy/organisational-development/swot-analysis-factsheet.

Earl. S., Carden. F. and Smutylo, T. (2001) *Outcome Mapping: Building Learning and Reflection into Development Programs*, International Development Research Centre, Canada.

Economics by Design (2020) *NHS Funded Library and Knowledge Services in England – Value Proposition: The Gift of Time*. www.hee.nhs.uk/our-work/library-knowledge-services/value-proposition-gift-time.

Foley, T. (2022) *The Role of Health Education England Knowledge and Library Services in Supporting Learning Health Systems*, Health Education England. https://library.nhs.uk/our-work/supporting-learning-health-systems.

Foley, T., Horowitz, L. and Zahran, R. (2021) *Realising the Potential of Learning Health Systems*, The Learning Healthcare Project, Health Foundation and Newcastle University. https://learninghealthcareproject.org/wp-content/uploads/2021/05/LHS2021report.pdf.

Health and Care Act 2022 (c31). www.legislation.gov.uk/ukpga/2022/31/introduction.

Health Education England (2021) *Knowledge for Healthcare: Mobilising Evidence; Sharing Knowledge; Improving Outcomes. A Strategic Framework for NHS Knowledge and Library Services 2021–26*. www.hee.nhs.uk/our-work/knowledge-for-healthcare.

Health Education England (2022) *Plan on a Page*. https://library.hee.nhs.uk/learning-academy/learning-zone/plan-on-a-page.

Kendrick, T. (2021) *Engaging your Community Through Active Strategic Marketing: A Practical Guide for Librarians and Information Professionals*, Facet Publishing.

National Health Library and Knowledge Service (2018) *Turning Knowledge Into Action: Enabling Care; Improving Health 2018–2023 – A Call to Collective Action for Users and Providers of Knowledge in the Health Service in Ireland*. www.lenus.ie/handle/10147/622955.

NHS Education for Scotland (2012) *Getting Knowledge Into Action to Improve Healthcare Quality: Report of Strategic Review and Recommendations*. https://learn.nes.nhs.scot/70279/finding-and-using-knowledge/about-knowledge-into-action/getting-knowledge-into-action-to-improve-healthcare-quality-report-of-strategic-review-and-recommendations.

NHS Education for Scotland (2016) *Knowledge Into Action in Scotland's Health and Social Services: Implementation of Knowledge Into Action 2013–2016*. https://learn.nes.nhs.scot/70280/finding-and-using-knowledge/about-knowledge-into-action/knowledge-into-action-in-scotland-s-health-and-social-services-implementation-of-knowledge-into-action-2013-2016.

NHS England and NHS Improvement (2022) *Online Library of Quality, Service Improvement and Redesign Tools: Driver Diagrams*. www.england.nhs.uk/wp-content/uploads/2022/01/qsir-driver-diagrams.pdf.

NHS Scotland (2022) *Delivering Value Based Health and Care: A Vision for Scotland*. www.gov.scot/publications/delivering-value-based-health-care-vision-scotland.

Roberts, S. and Rowley, J. (2008) *Leadership: The Challenge for the Information Profession*, Facet Publishing.

SCONUL (2023) *Key Performance Indicators*. www.sconul.ac.uk/page/key-performance-indicators.

Showers, B. (2015) *Library Analytics and Metrics: Using Data to Drive Decisions and Services*, Facet Publishing.

3

Exploring the Training and Development Needs of the Healthcare Knowledge and Library Services Workforce: A Case Study

Dominic Gilroy and Catherine McLaren

Introduction

Most employers recognise that the workforce is the most important asset of the organisation. This is certainly true within healthcare knowledge and library services where evidence has repeatedly illustrated the economic benefit that this staff group bring to the NHS by releasing time for busy healthcare professionals (Economics by Design, 2020).

To perform efficiently and to cater for the evolving needs of healthcare, it is crucial that the workforce has opportunities to develop and expand their skills. Often, the provision of training and development are seen as an easy target when funds are short. False economies are made by cutting back on training and development opportunities that leave the workforce with less of the crucial knowledge and skills needed to help the organisation develop (Kumar, 2015, 16). By contrast, a recent European study (Dietz and Zwick, 2020, 712) found that credible training and development opportunities can increase retention rates by up to 18%.

As steward of NHS knowledge and library services in England, Health Education England (HEE) hold the remit for the provision of learning and development for the knowledge and library services workforce. This chapter outlines HEE's approach to identifying, planning and delivering the training and development needs of the healthcare knowledge and library services workforce. Although these interventions are described in the context of HEE, the reader will note that many of the approaches are generic and may be transferrable to similar contexts elsewhere.

For the avoidance of doubt, it should be noted that this chapter focuses on exploring the needs of the knowledge and library workforce rather than the needs of service users and customers.

Establishing routes into the sector

The training and development needs of the healthcare knowledge and library services workforce begin before they take up their roles within healthcare libraries. Future members of the workforce need an awareness of the sector and an insight into the roles and types of work undertaken by healthcare knowledge and library specialists. This awareness and knowledge is essential, not least because it sparks an interest in work within healthcare and prompts applications for posts.

HEE has taken a proactive approach to promoting roles in healthcare knowledge and library services at a number of different levels.

Higher education institutions

Knowledge and library specialists working in professional roles within healthcare will often hold a CILIP accredited master's degree in a knowledge, library and information related subject. HEE's national knowledge and library team has engaged with each of the higher education institutions offering these CILIP accredited courses based in England to ensure there is a health-related presence on these courses. This varies from a recorded session or live lecture as part of the curriculum, to a full healthcare libraries module, such as those that have been delivered at Manchester Metropolitan University and University College London. In addition to providing a general overview of the themes of healthcare library work, these modules include a focus on priorities within the sector, including knowledge mobilisation, health literacy, embedded librarianship and quality and impact.

This presence on educational courses ensures that future professionals have an awareness of healthcare knowledge and library services as a potential future career. It also better prepares those entering the profession in terms of what to expect from healthcare knowledge roles.

Apprenticeships

Apprenticeships can be popular with employees as a means of learning on the job while earning a wage. Apprentices develop and learn while undertaking a paid role. By the end of the apprenticeship, they will have the correct mix of knowledge and skills, as well as experience, to progress in their chosen career.

Apprenticeships are an increasingly common form of employment in NHS organisations since the UK government places an apprenticeship levy of 0.5% on all organisations with a pay bill of £3 million or above per annum. Organisations are then able to recover these costs by employing apprentices.

HEE has worked with CILIP on the introduction of a Level 3 Apprenticeship for Museums, Libraries and Archives (Institute for Apprenticeships and Technical Education, 2022), with apprentices employed in a range of NHS knowledge and library services. HEE is also part of a trailblazer group pursuing a Level 6/7 apprenticeship for the profession. Once available, it is anticipated this will provide another route for knowledge specialists to join healthcare services.

NHS Health Careers

NHS Health Careers is a careers advice platform providing an insight into the vast range of careers available within the NHS and healthcare.

HEE has worked with NHS Health Careers to ensure that knowledge and library roles are included in this package (NHS Health Careers, 2022). The site provides an overview of NHS knowledge and library work and signposts to current vacancies within the profession. It includes some recent case studies of real-life knowledge and library staff and their career profiles and current jobs to provide an insight into actual roles in NHS knowledge and library services.

Identifying development needs

When considering learning and development needs it is important to be clear about the intended recipients. Who is the learning targeted at and who is eligible to attend? A second consideration is whether there are any specific types of learning that need to be prioritised. Are there strategically important skills and learning that need to be included?

We will look at each of these areas in turn and provide some examples from the work of HEE's knowledge and library team to illustrate possible approaches.

Workforce coverage

The title of this chapter indicates that the intended recipients of our learning are the 'healthcare knowledge and library services workforce'. When considering the planning and development of the learning, it is important to consider the range of specific groups within this broader workforce. For example, is the learning aimed at the workforce within a particular country or geographical area? Is it aimed at the workforce of a specific employer? Is the learning aimed at a particular staff group or role, for example, library managers or library assistants? There may be other considerations that should be taken into account in a particular circumstance or situation.

In the case of HEE, its geographical area of coverage is, unsurprisingly, England. It is primarily concerned with providing learning and development opportunities to NHS funded knowledge and library specialists. This includes those members of the workforce directly employed by the NHS or those employed by organisations providing knowledge and library services to the NHS under a funded service level agreement. Learning is usually extended to colleagues working in organisations such as Public Health, Royal Colleges, hospices, charities and NHS Arm's Length Bodies. In addition, HEE is increasingly working across national borders with colleagues in other UK home nations, with online learning extended to these colleagues.

In terms of the job roles covered, our remit is to provide learning and development opportunities for the full knowledge and library specialist team from apprentices, library assistants and paraprofessionals through to more senior library managers.

Types of learning needs

Defining the parameters of the learning needs to be addressed is an important step in the process. An individual may have personal aspirations to develop in a range of different areas unrelated to their job role but many of these are likely to fall outside the remit of the learning provider. It is particularly prudent to consider broader strategic requirements when prioritising learning provision. If the driver for the provision of learning and develop opportunities is the achievement of specific strategic aims and objectives, then the choice of opportunities developed should enable staff to develop skills and knowledge that will help to achieve these goals.

From the perspective of HEE, we are interested in learning needs that are knowledge and library service related and associated with the individual's employment within healthcare. In particular, there is a prioritisation of learning requirements that are associated with our national Knowledge for Healthcare strategy (Health Education England, 2021) or aimed at service improvement and aligned with the NHS Knowledge and Library Services Quality and Improvement Outcomes Framework (Health Education England, 2019), the local quality assurance processes for NHS healthcare libraries in England. This ensures that our limited resources are targeted effectively.

Funding

In cases where learning and development opportunities are being provided for colleagues from multiple organisations by a central body, finances are a crucial consideration. What funding is available and where does that funding come from? A number of models could be considered, including:

- self-funded courses where individuals, or their employer, pay for attendance on an individual case-by-case basis
- Levy model where organisations pay an annual fee for their members to be eligible to attend an event or range of events
- centrally funded courses where an organisation commissions and funds a learning offer for the workforce.

The third model, adopted by HEE for the healthcare knowledge and library services workforce, has advantages in that it allows an organisation to tailor learning closely to the needs of the workforce. There is more likelihood of equity of access across the system since delegates are not expected to self-fund and their involvement is accepted or even expected by managers and the organisation. There is less dependence on the availability and prioritisation of local budgets.

Within an NHS environment there would be little likelihood of individual NHS trusts arranging learning and development opportunities for their knowledge and library staff. The challenge is due in part to the very small number of knowledge and library specialists working in individual organisations. While it may be cost efficient to fund an internal course for 300 nurses, it is unlikely to be considered viable to run an event for four or five library staff.

HEE steps in to fill this gap for the NHS knowledge and library workforce. Our NHS Knowledge for Healthcare Learning Academy has a remit to provide a range of learning opportunities for the healthcare knowledge and library workforce in England (Gilroy and Smith, 2022).

Development needs survey

Knowledge and library specialists, like all service providers, know the importance of user consultation in developing service provision. It is essential to consider the opinions and requests of the knowledge and library workforce when planning and developing learning:

> Training needs analysis is the initial step in a cyclical process which contributes to the overall training and educational strategy of staff in an organisation or a professional group. The cycle commences with a systematic consultation to identify the learning needs of the population considered, followed by course planning, delivery and evaluation.
>
> (Gould, 2004, 471)

The term 'development needs analysis' is preferred within HEE's knowledge and library team as we recognise that learning needs extend beyond traditional training and education and may be addressed through a broad range of interventions.

HEE's main means of regular consultation with our knowledge and library workforce is through the biennial Workforce Planning and Development Survey, which incorporates a development needs survey. The survey is anonymous and aimed at all healthcare knowledge and library staff in England. It is made available online for participants and advertised through a range of our regular communication channels, with participants usually being allowed one month to respond.

McLelland (1994, 22) identifies four advantages of survey questionnaires over other forms of research. The first relates to the fact that, compared to some other methods, they provide a means to gather input from a wide range of people over a large geographical location without the need for travel and the associated costs and inconvenience. Secondly, they are less intrusive than other forms of research, thus reducing stress for participants. Thirdly, they are less open to the bias that can occur in smaller numbers of interviews with individuals. Finally, they are relatively quick and simple for participants to complete. We might add that the anonymity provided by online surveys may encourage delegates to be more truthful in their responses, particularly if they have constructive criticism they wish to share.

The response rate is always an important consideration when undertaking surveys. When basing decisions on the results of the development needs survey, it is important for the response rate to be as high as possible and to be representative of all areas of the workforce.

While a 100% response rate may be desirable, it is also an unrealistic expectation. Baruch and Holtom (2008, 1139) looked at 490 surveys published between 2000 and 2005 and identified an average response rate of 52.7%. They also noted a steady decline in response rates over the years and hypothesised that this decline would continue.

HEE's Development Needs Survey response rate is usually slightly higher than this average. In 2019, there was around a 56% response, although the response rate for 2021 fell dramatically for a range of reasons, not least of which being the distraction of the pandemic. In addition, the survey responses usually include good representation from the library manager, knowledge and library specialist and library assistant/paraprofessional areas of the workforce.

Precision of requirements

The translation of requests flagged by a development needs survey into tangible learning can be challenging. The themes emerging from the development needs analysis are sometimes too vague to be worked into a specific training course, e-learning offering or electronic resource without further investigation.

One route to avoid this is to offer specific options within the development needs survey to ensure clarity at the analysis stage. It is also possible to undertake further analysis of any emerging themes using interviews, focus groups or through approaching workforce representatives. This helps develop a clearer understanding of the need so that interventions can be focused accordingly.

Two examples of this from HEE's 2019 Development Needs Survey are Emerging Technologies and Critical Appraisal:

- Emerging Technologies was chosen as one of the top four themes for all four of the staff groups and was the top theme for Band 5 (entry level qualified librarians) and Band 7 plus (library managers). It is a theme that does not lend itself easily to interpretation in terms of a learning and development intervention and further work needed to be done before associated learning could be made available.
- Critical appraisal skills, while a little more specific, are also a fairly vague concept in a knowledge and library specialist domain. It was unclear whether respondents were interested in beginner level introductory courses, more advanced training on the appraisal of specific types of study (qualitative, quantitative, Randomised Controlled Trials, Systematic Reviews) or train the trainer offerings designed to equip delegates with the skills to facilitate critical appraisal training sessions themselves. Further work was required to refine the needs before learning could be put in place.

Focus groups and interviews

While widespread surveys of the workforce can be useful in determining the breadth of learning and development needs, it can be helpful to supplement this approach with a more personal engagement with key groups.

Sava (2012, 70–1) notes that focus groups can be particularly useful for exploring people's knowledge and experience and examine not only what participants' views are but also the rationale behind these views. Consequently, they are particularly useful as a tool to investigate the nuances of specific problems and needs.

HEE took this approach when determining the development and learning needs of new and aspiring managers within the NHS knowledge and library workforce. A decline in the number of applicants for manager roles over several years was identified by members of HEE's knowledge and library team who work closely with organisations in support of recruitment. Initial investigations suggested that the low numbers of applicants may be due in part to confidence and skills gaps among potential applicants.

In response, HEE arranged focus groups with current and aspiring knowledge and library managers and interviewed several line managers responsible for recruiting knowledge and library managers with the aim of understanding the skills, experience and knowledge an individual needs to be successful in the role. This was followed by an analysis of how HEE could work with individuals and organisations to develop new and aspiring managers through a range of interventions. In response, a learning package was created to support new and aspiring managers to develop an interest in, and apply for, these roles.

Expert input

The role of senior stakeholders, specialist interest groups (SIGs) and subject matter experts (SMEs) is also important in the planning and development of learning opportunities. The contribution of senior stakeholders and decision makers is important as they can often help align learning plans with organisational goals.

Specialist interest groups, especially where they consist of representatives of the workforce who will participate in the learning, can also provide an invaluable perspective. Such groups might include specialists in a particular field, such as clinical librarians, information skills trainers or library assistants, who gather to share good practice and offer peer support. Members of such groups will often be senior and/or experienced colleagues able to speak formally or informally on behalf of the workforce or groups within it.

Subject matter experts are also a valuable resource. In the arena of knowledge and library services, these experts will often be practitioners in the field and be able to bring their expertise and experience to bear in planning and developing learning opportunities for colleagues.

HEE's Knowledge and Library Services Workforce Planning and Development Steering Group has been essential in the planning and development of learning for the health knowledge and library workforce. The steering group includes representation from CILIP, higher education institutions (including schools of library and information science), knowledge managers and colleagues from all levels of the knowledge and library workforce. It provides a sounding board for advice and ideas relating to workforce planning and development, including learning opportunities.

Several SIGs regularly feed into the planning of HEE's learning and development opportunities for the knowledge and library workforce. Groups with an interest in continuing professional development exist throughout England, sometimes as part of formal networks, such as the well established

Library and Information Health Network Northwest (LIHHN – www.lksnorth.nhs.uk/lihnn). These groups play an important role in highlighting learning and development needs that may have been missed by the development needs survey and other routes. They act as voices for the wider workforce and are an essential element in the overall planning of opportunities.

Quality assurance in learning provision – The NHS Knowledge for Healthcare Learning Academy

In providing learning opportunities for the specialist healthcare knowledge and library workforce, the importance of quality assurance should not be underestimated. It is important to demonstrate the quality of the learning both to learners themselves, who are being invited to register and engage with the learning, but also to managers and employers who are releasing staff to attend learning and development courses.

Clarity about the content of courses, and its relevance to the profession and the sector in which the learner is working, is one aspect of this assurance. This can be achieved by demonstrating the relevance of the learning outcomes to the needs of the learner and the profession. Another important factor is the credentials, experience and expertise of the course facilitator or trainer. Recognised experts, experienced in the field, attract learners to participate.

Accreditation by an external body can bring these and other factors together to enhance the value of the learning on offer.

HEE's NHS Knowledge for Healthcare Learning Academy was developed with these considerations in mind (Gilroy and Smith, 2022). Our short-course learning offerings are accredited by CILIP, providing assurance to employers and learners that the learning has been assessed by a well established and respected professional body independent of HEE. The accreditation process reviews the processes and procedures in use within HEE for the development and delivery of learning opportunities. There is a review of the credentials and experience of the various facilitators and trainers delivering the learning and each course is mapped to CILIP's Professional Knowledge and Skills Base (PKSB) to demonstrate its relevance to the profession.

Responding to changing priorities – COVID-19

COVID-19 was declared a global pandemic by the World Health Organization on 11 March 2020 (World Health Organization, 2022) and placed substantial strain on the health and social care systems across the world, including in England. On 20 March 2020, the UK went into lockdown. Throughout this period, HEE continued to maintain the development and training opportunities available to the healthcare knowledge and library services workforce.

As we have seen earlier, formal development and training opportunities for knowledge and library service staff supported by HEE is always an evolving and continuous process based on the development needs survey, focus groups, interviews and expert input. While it is important to have plans in place in relation to learning and development, it is also vital that the provider, in this case HEE, can be flexible and respond to emerging trends, priorities and emergencies.

The COVID-19 pandemic was an emergency that led to fast moving changes to priorities. As NHS organisations responded to the needs of the pandemic in March 2020, many knowledge and library staff working in healthcare found themselves redeployed at short notice, with others asked to work from home. HEE's face-to-face training for this staff group was put on hold or cancelled as a result.

Online learning

While traditional face-to-face training and development was postponed, or eventually cancelled, virtual learning and online webinars emerged as a solution to meet the needs of this small specialist workforce. Much of the NHS workforce had their education changed in a similar way. A recent review on the effects of the pandemic on medical education showed that online learning was the most frequent method used to mitigate the COVID-19 challenges (Chasset et al., 2022).

Online sessions offer several advantages: they are easily accessible; often much cheaper to run due to the absence of room hire, hotel or transport costs; and are easier to repeat so that more people can access the opportunity. When sessions are recorded, people can access the learning at a time convenient for them or go back and review the learning after the live sessions.

We chose to focus on two key areas in the early phase of the pandemic – how to use virtual sessions to deliver knowledge and library services and supporting the health and wellbeing of the staff.

Virtual training

HEE's initial focus during the pandemic was on ensuring that knowledge and library service staff were equipped with the skills to facilitate meetings and training sessions online. The intention was to provide opportunities for the knowledge and library workforce to get to grips with the technology and learn some of the tips and tricks for getting the most out of virtual sessions. Time was given to thinking about the tools available for managing and facilitating face-to-face meetings and transferring them to the virtual environment.

Working with a trainer external to HEE, a three-hour session was developed on the theme of 'facilitating virtual meetings'. This session focused on four key areas:

1 Meeting our objectives
2 Keeping people engaged
3 Making good decisions
4 Staying efficient.

This list can work for any meeting, but the session really focused on how this worked in the virtual environment. A second session was then developed to focus in more detail on how to deliver training online. In the five months between May 2020 and September 2020, over 110 NHS knowledge and library staff attended this training.

Health and wellbeing

Anecdotal evidence quickly established that some knowledge and library staff were struggling in the early part of the pandemic. In some cases, knowledge and library services closed and staff were redeployed into other roles, some of them to the frontline. Many knowledge and library staff were informed that their services needed to be delivered virtually and were instructed to work from home. Others provided some form of face-to-face service with varying levels of restrictions and social distancing in place. All staff were facing an unknown scenario with uncertainty in terms of what the future would bring. These findings match the findings for much larger staff groups within the NHS.

Levels of burnout among nurses and midwives have been reported to be higher in the UK than in other countries, with UK nurses and midwives reporting higher levels of mental health problems, such as depression and anxiety, compared to the general working population (Hunter et al., 2019; Kinman, Teoh and Harriss, 2020, 17). Other health and social care occupations in the UK, such as social workers, were also reported to be experiencing high levels of work-related stress (McFadden, Mallett and Leiter, 2018, 72; Ravalier et al., 2020, 1105). The added pressures of COVID-19 put the health and social care workforce, including knowledge and library staff, under even more strain and led to more stress and potentially lower wellbeing. HEE wanted to support and equip staff and their teams to cope with the ongoing situation.

In response to this concern, sessions were developed in four areas covering the health and wellbeing needs of healthcare knowledge and library staff during the pandemic:

1 Looking after yourself: personal resilience while working remotely
2 Looking after others: supporting colleagues 1-1
3 Leading remote teams in a pandemic; fostering resilience
4 Leading remote teams.

If these sessions had been face-to-face, there may have been between 20 and 40 people interested and able to attend from across England. By delivering the sessions virtually, it was possible to offer 180 places across the four sessions and considerable interest was demonstrated by the workforce. The vast increase in demand for these virtual learning opportunities was a recurring theme throughout the pandemic, with the team struggling to meet demand and often needing to repeat courses several times to cater for the numbers interested.

Needs of different staff groups

Several distinct staff groups exist within the wider NHS knowledge and library workforce. When thinking about the development needs of these groups, some subject areas are consistent for all staff, while others have specific development needs relating to their roles. There are three particular groups of staff where some bespoke learning and development opportunities are offered.

Paraprofessional or library assistant staff

As some of the administrative activities undertaken by this group of staff are similar to other administrative roles within NHS organisations, it is sometimes the case that this group of staff have been able to access development opportunities within their own organisations. These opportunities might include customer service and/or business administration apprenticeships and training. These opportunities rarely cover the knowledge and library specialism within their role, meaning that there is still a need for specialist knowledge and library service learning and development opportunities.

In line with the general trend of a move to virtual learning, development opportunities for this group of staff have moved online over the last few years. Tailored local library assistant study days, which once attracted 15 or so colleagues as a face-to-face event, moved online in 2020, attracting over

50 staff from across England in the first year and 200 in 2021. Topics covered over the years include: career development; using social media; sharing and solving problems; creating displays; writing for good copy; searching the deep web; developing enquiry skills; and accessibility.

Paraprofessional staff are also able to access the more general knowledge and library services training and development opportunities provided by HEE. A number of sessions are developed to be useful to all staffing groups within NHS knowledge and library services. These include: health literacy sessions; social media and marketing training; and health and wellbeing sessions.

Clinical and embedded librarians

Clinical and embedded librarians have enjoyed a range of training and development opportunities developed independently of HEE. There are several regional communities of practice and email discussion lists organised and managed by interested individuals. The International Clinical Librarian Conference (University Hospitals of Leicester NHS Trust, 2021), organised by the University Hospitals of Leicester Clinical Librarian Service, is a key offer for this group of staff. The event gathers a national and international audience of clinical and embedded librarians and knowledge specialists to look at the latest research and share developments from across the world. HEE has worked in partnership with the organisers to support the event over the years and in 2021 provided administrative and technical support to the conference team so that a shortened programme was able to go ahead virtually.

HEE also provides a range of other specialist training sessions that will be of particular interest to clinical and embedded librarians and knowledge specialists. These include courses covering critical appraisal, summarising and synthesising, and expert searching skills.

Knowledge and library service managers

Over recent years, HEE has been developing the support and training offered to knowledge and library service managers. One area of focus has been around a Senior Leadership Development Programme. This programme runs over six or nine months. It is targeted at senior healthcare librarians and knowledge specialists who are already leading a service, team or network and who wish to strengthen their effectiveness as leaders. The programme is designed to benefit individuals with a minimum of three years' leadership experience who want to make a difference through their work, reach their full potential, widen their portfolios and shape their career. It involves a series of workshops, action learning sets and coaching sessions. It focuses on developing strategic leadership skills, leading inclusively, managing change and leading across and within systems. The programme includes participating in a group project to help progress the ambitions of national Knowledge for Healthcare (Health Education England, 2021).

Additional opportunities are being developed to support knowledge and library service managers, including those new in post. Members of the HEE knowledge and library services team meet with new managers to discuss recommended training, relevant national and local information and HEE quality processes. These meetings continue in the short and medium term, depending on the needs of the manager. The meetings cover areas such as agreeing goals, identifying development needs and building a relationship between the manager and HEE. Mentoring, buddying or coaching for the new manager are also available depending on individual requirements.

It is anticipated that managers will continue to develop their skills throughout their career and they are encouraged to continue to access the range of learning and development opportunities offered by HEE, including the senior leadership development programme mentioned above. Regional managers' meetings offer additional ongoing support from both HEE and peers. These meetings take place several times a year and enable managers to meet together to discuss issues, hear from speakers, share good practice and learn from each other. There is also an opportunity to hear updates from and ask questions of the HEE national knowledge and library services team. Lunchtime learning sessions on a range of relevant topics, open to existing and aspiring managers, launched in 2022 and randomised coffee trials have also been developed. These offer opportunities for a short virtual conversation between an experienced and aspiring manager to help generate interest and knowledge of what the role involves.

Professional staff

The focus on the three particular staff groups above does not mean that other professional knowledge and library service staff do not have access to training and development opportunities. There is a wide range of opportunities available to the whole NHS knowledge and library workforce and it is key that staff access these opportunities. Many staff embarking on their careers in healthcare libraries will go on to be either clinical and embedded librarians or managers later in their career. In anticipation of this, a Leadership Development Programme, aimed at less senior staff, relaunched in 2022. The programme is tailored for healthcare knowledge and library specialists. It is not just for those with formal management responsibility, but is also aimed at people who wish to develop and strengthen their effectiveness as they take on a variety of leadership roles. It is focused on individuals who have some leadership experience and early career managers who are looking to build on their skills for the future.

Conclusion

This chapter has explored the HEE knowledge and library services team's approach to the identification of the training and development needs of current and future healthcare knowledge and library staff and how these have been developed into specific targeted offerings for the workforce.

It explores some of the challenges encountered in delivering this work and covers the response to ever changing priorities within healthcare, including how learning was tailored to online delivery during the COVID pandemic.

Although focused on healthcare knowledge and library services in England, it is anticipated that many of these approaches will be relevant and transferrable to healthcare systems in other countries.

References

Baruch, Y. and Holtom, B. (2008) Survey Response Rate Levels and Trends in Organizational Research, *Human Relations*, **61** (8), 1139–60.

Chasset, F., Barral, M., Steichen, O. and Legrand, A. (2022) Immediate Consequences and Solutions Used to Maintain Medical Education During the Covid-19 Pandemic for Residents and Medical Students: A Restricted Review, *Postgraduate Medical Journal*, **98** (1159), 380–8.

Dietz, D. and Zwick, T. (2020) The Retention Effect of Training: Portability, Visibility, and Credibility, *The International Journal of Human Resource Management*, **33** (4), 710–41.

Economics by Design (2020) *NHS Funded Library and Knowledge Services in England – Value Proposition: The Gift of Time*. www.hee.nhs.uk/our-work/library-knowledge-services/value-proposition-gift-time.

Gilroy, D. and Smith, S. (2022) Accredited Informatics Skills Development Opportunities for the NHS Knowledge and Library Specialist Workforce in England. In Scott, P., Mantas, J., Benis, A., Ognjanovic, I., Saranto, A., Wells, I. and Gallos, P. (eds), *Digital Professionalism in Health and Care: Developing the Workforce, Building the Future*, 13–18, IOS Press. https://ebooks.iospress.nl/volumearticle/60668.

Gould, D., Kelly, D., White, I. and Chidgey, J. (2004) Training Needs Analysis. A Literature Review and Reappraisal. *International Journal of Nursing Studies*, **41** (5), 471–86.

Health Education England (2019) Quality and Improvement Outcomes Framework for NHS Funded Library and Knowledge Services in England, www.hee.nhs.uk/sites/default/files/documents/HEE%20Quality%20and%20Improvement%20Outcomes%20Framework.pdf.

Health Education England (2021) Knowledge for Healthcare: Mobilising
   Evidence; Sharing Knowledge; Improving Outcomes. *A Strategic
   Framework for NHS Knowledge and Library Services 2021–2026.*
   www.hee.nhs.uk/sites/default/files/documents/HEE%20Knowledge%20for
   %20Healthcare%202021-26%20FINAL.pdf.
Hunter, B., Fenwick, J., Sidebotham, M. and Henley, J. (2019) Midwives in
   the United Kingdom: Levels of Burnout, Depression, Anxiety and Stress
   and Associated Predictors, *Midwifery*, 79, 1–12.
Institute for Apprenticeships and Technical Education (2022) Library,
   Information and Archives Services Assistant.
   www.cilip.org.uk/page/LISApprenticeships.
Kinman, G., Teoh, K. and Harriss, A. (2020) *The Mental Health and Wellbeing
   of Nurses and Midwives in the United Kingdom*, Society of Occupational
   Medicine. www.som.org.uk/sites/som.org.uk/files/The_Mental_Health_
   and_Wellbeing_of_Nurses_and_Midwives_in_the_United_Kingdom.pdf.
Kumar, D. (2015) Strategic HR Initiatives to Combat Economic Recession,
   Review of Professional Management, 7 (1), 12–21.
McFadden, P., Mallett, J. and Leiter, M. (2018) Extending the Two-Process
   Model of Burnout in Child Protection Workers: The Role of Resilience in
   Mediating Burnout Via Organizational Factors of Control, Values, Fairness,
   Reward, Workload, and Community Relationship, *Stress Health*, 34 (1),
   72–83.
McLelland, S. (1994) Training Needs Assessment Data-Gathering Methods:
   Part 1, Survey Questionnaires, *Journal of European Industrial Training*, 18
   (1), 22–7.
NHS Health Careers (2022) Knowledge and Library Services.
   www.healthcareers.nhs.uk/explore-roles/health-informatics/roles-health-
   informatics/knowledge-and-library-services.
Ravalier, J., Wainwright, E., Clabburn, O. and Loon, M. (2021) Working
   Conditions and Wellbeing in UK Social Workers, *Journal of Social Work*, 21
   (5), 1105–23.
Sava, S. (2012) Methods of Needs Analysis in Educational Context. In Sava,
   S. (ed), *Needs Analysis and Programme Planning in Adult Education*, 59–
   88, Barbara Budrich Publishers.
University Hospitals of Leicester NHS Trust (2021) *ICLC International
   Clinical Librarian Conference*. www.uhl-library.nhs.uk/iclc/index.html.
World Health Organization (2022) *Coronavirus Disease (COVID-19)
   Pandemic*. www.who.int/europe/emergencies/situations/covid-19.

4

Advocacy and How Knowledge and Library Specialists Tailor Services to Meet the Needs of Their Stakeholders

Holly Case Wyatt

Special thanks to Vicky Bramwell, Library Services Manager at Cheshire and Wirral Partnership NHS Foundation Trust, for her contribution to this chapter.

Introduction

The learning outcomes in this chapter include a greater understanding of advocacy as a skill that all knowledge and library staff should utilise to promote and develop their service; the importance of identifying key stakeholders and understanding their needs; and how advocacy skills can be nurtured in knowledge and library specialists.

This chapter will explore the importance of advocacy for knowledge and library staff working in healthcare and how health knowledge and library specialists can use their advocacy skills to tailor services for stakeholders. In healthcare knowledge and library services, the need to advocate for services, skills and space is linked to the large, changeable organisations and workforces they serve.

Most knowledge and library specialists working in a health service will have had to defend their service at some point in their career. This may have been in relation to the need for physical or electronic stock, for an appropriate budget, a suitable space and, in some extreme examples, the existence of the entire service. However, the advocacy undertaken in health knowledge and library services also incorporates an element of selling and promotion and many knowledge and library specialists will have developed an internal script they use to sell their services – for example, by showcasing the electronic resources that will benefit the particular person they are speaking to. It is a skill to know what you can use to tempt a new service user, for example, timely current awareness bulletins, time-saving searches or help with a journal club. There is an element of intuitiveness in understanding your service users' needs, but work should also be undertaken to map your service users and their potential needs for more effective promotion and for service development. Often, the advocacy and promotional activities undertaken lead to the enhancement of essential library services for healthcare staff.

The case studies throughout this chapter will showcase how different knowledge and library services in England have been able to advocate elements of their provision to new groups and then tailor their services to them. A number of themes emerge showing that advocacy in the right situations and circumstances can lead to successful projects and engagement from wider groups. Almost all case studies show that one project will often snowball and lead to further engagement with new service users.

For many knowledge and library specialists, advocacy is an intuitive part of the profession or something that is learnt on the job. Although once not considered part of the traditional skill set of a librarian, advocacy is now seen as an essential aspect of the profession. It is 'an obligation, a necessity, and the core of a librarian's role' (Hicks, 2016, 625). Advocacy has been particularly identified as an important part of information literacy in higher education. Secker and Walton (2015) suggest it is central to 'raising awareness, understanding that language and terminology [of information literacy] matter and in making explicit the links between information literacy and stakeholders' priorities'. In CILIP's Professional Knowledge and Skills Base (PKSB), advocacy is included under the 'Generic Skills' section, within *Leadership, Advocacy, Influencing and Personal Effectiveness*. CILIP defines advocacy as:

> … building relationships to facilitate strategic advantage. Managing a professional profile to increase opportunities to engage and network. Securing opportunities to increase engagement with key messages from target audiences.
>
> (CILIP, 2022)

This encourages all knowledge and library specialists undertaking professional registration or revalidation to reflect on their advocacy skills within their work.

Institutions offering CILIP accredited library and information management studies are including advocacy as part of their curriculum for their students. On University College London's Information Studies postgraduate programme, advocacy is included in a number of modules, including *Managing Information Organisations* and the *Library and Information Professional* (UCL, 2022). This sets their students up to start thinking about the role of advocacy in their professional working lives from the beginning, particularly when linked to strategic thinking, leadership and influencing skills. Manchester Metropolitan University's Master's in Library and Information Management programme includes advocacy as part of

Information Organisations and their Management. This unit enables students to comprehend and analyse how the PKSB describes the way in which librarians and information professionals might apply the notion of advocacy in their professional role.

It is important to acknowledge the link between advocacy, promotion and marketing, all essential tools for a knowledge and library specialist. Advocacy is often considered a continuum with marketing and promotion (Hicks, 2016, 617) and we see opportunities for knowledge and library specialists to advocate during a promotional activity or following on from marketing services. It is important to understand and acknowledge the link between advocacy, marketing and promotion, however, they are separate activities that need different skill sets.

How are librarians advocating?

Already underpinning knowledge and library services are general services for users that we might describe as 'traditional' services. These services, such as study space and evidence searching, are still major selling points in advocacy. Whilst offering evidence searching is not specifically tailoring knowledge and library services to your users, there is also an understanding, for example, that we would not offer an evidence search to anyone undertaking a study course as this should be a skill developed as part of their learning. We instead offer a 'finding the evidence' training session so that the service user can undertake their own literature searching. This is one small example of how knowledge and library specialists tweak services based on specific user need. Knowledge of the 'traditional' services on offer, for example, journals, electronic resources, exam resources and current awareness, is essential for all knowledge and library specialists. This allows you to have an arsenal of selling points available to use at any time for all current and potential service users. To maximise this opportunity, it is useful to research your potential audience before meeting them, or even ask their role when you meet, so that tailored conversations can happen.

Saving time for our users has long been a promotional tool used by knowledge and library specialists to advocate for our involvement with projects and working groups. When positioned at the right time, our 'traditional' services, such as evidence searching and current awareness, can be a tool to support time saving. As long as the group you are working with already understands the need for evidence within their work, showing them how you can save their time and therefore increase productivity can often be the most important piece in your advocacy puzzle. Case Study 4.1 below highlights the work of an embedded librarian in a community trust.

Case Study 4.1: Embedded knowledge specialist attends a multi-disciplinary team (MDT)

Team/project lead: NHS East Dorset Knowledge and Library Service / Su Keill

Trust: Dorset Healthcare University NHS Foundation Trust

Target group: A post-COVID syndrome multi-disciplinary team (MDT)

Following holding a focus group for library users where it was mentioned that knowledge and library specialists could attend MDT meetings to support with evidence, the librarian was invited to be part of a newly set up county-wide MDT to deal with patients being referred with post-COVID syndrome. As this initial invitation came from the chronic fatigue syndrome/ME Lead at the Community Trust who was a frequent user of the service, there was already an in-built champion within the team who could steer how the librarian was utilised. This topic is still very new and under constant review, which means that the librarian was able to provide resources and evidence directly at meetings, take away literature searches and provide examples of other organisations undertaking similar work. As research was found, it was added onto a platform so that any new starters would have access to it. Recently, the knowledge and library specialist has been asked to write plain-English patient information on post-COVID syndrome, including summaries and links. As there are a range of health professionals from across three trusts in the county, including GPs and Allied Health Professionals, it also acts as a promotional tool for the service.

Key themes: relationship building, seizing an opportunity, highlighting services and skills

---

Whilst attendance at an MDT is not new or unusual for a knowledge and library specialist in an embedded, clinical, outreach or similar role, this Case Study 4.1 highlights a number of important advocacy themes. In trying to further their understanding of the service user, the knowledge and library service has utilised a focus group, which has then led to this opportunity. Often, we see opportunities such as this one arise from a knowledge and library specialist advocating for the service in a different situation or promotional activity. Already having a library user within the MDT has minimised the need for advocating for evidence as an intrinsic part of patient care, which has been embedded since the instigation of the group. Most importantly, we can see the clear progression of the group's understanding of the skills and services that their embedded knowledge and library specialist can offer. From 'traditional' services, such as providing evidence and literature searches, they are now supporting the production of high quality, evidence-based patient information.

Relationship building is an integral part of advocacy for healthcare knowledge and library services. Being able to identify a meaningful commonality (Cialdini, Wissler and Schweitzer, 2002, 20) with the person or group to whom you are advocating may increase your chances of positively influencing them. Whilst advocating for knowledge and library services, you will need to consider how you articulate your services so that the stakeholder can relate it to their own goals, sometimes even pre-emptively before they have explicitly stated those goals to you. In healthcare environments, we all share a common goal in wanting to achieve the best outcomes for patients, which may be an easy way to link your common goals together. Other commonalities to explore include time saving, money saving and innovations, all of which are key priorities within the NHS as well as most other organisations and institutions. Also, not forgetting upskilling the healthcare workforce, this enables organisations to fill roles where demand is great or build research confidence so that they become more research active, implementing research and sharing outputs. Knowledge and library specialists should be asking themselves: what does my stakeholder want to achieve and how can I help them do that?

It is good practice to ensure that your knowledge and library service strategy is aligned to both the national priorities laid out by your overarching body (such as NHS England in England) and those of your organisation. Strategic alignment to both sets of priorities will show how your services contribute to supporting the success of your organisation (HEE, 2021) and act as a roadmap for service development. This is another example of showcasing a shared goal. Case Study 4.2 below exemplifies how a knowledge and library service was able to determine how it could support a key priority of its trust and which services would add to the value of it.

Case Study 4.2: Embedding library and knowledge services in the quality improvement process

Team/project lead: Gloucestershire Hospitals Library and Knowledge Service / Lisa Riddington

Trust: Gloucestershire Hospitals NHS Foundation Trust

Target group: The Quality Improvement Team at Gloucestershire Hospitals

When the Library and Knowledge Services (LKS) Manager at Gloucestershire Hospitals NHS Foundation Trust initially met with the lead developing the Quality Improvement (QI) Academy to discuss how the library might enable the success of the Academy and embed evidence into the QI process, the Academy decided that a leaflet about the library in all project folders would be sufficient. Whilst initially disappointed, the LKS team agreed and continued to seek opportunities.

The LKS Manager attended a QI Silver Project Level Graduation event where a junior doctor told her how they had found the information for their QI project via Google and how if they'd had help from the library it would have been beneficial. Using this information, the LKS team managed to secure a five-minute slot on a teaching session to talk about literature searching to all those undertaking a new QI project. But the real turning point for the involvement of LKS came when the LKS Manager undertook her own Silver Award QI project and the rest of the LKS Team attended the Bronze Award. This not only gave the team an opportunity to expand their understanding of the Academy and QI in general, but they were also able to network and promote the LKS service.

Throughout this relationship building, the LKS team bided their time until the QI team recognised that LKS should be embedded right at the start of the QI project process. Now all those undertaking a QI project in the Trust are signposted to the LKS, the LKS Manager is part of the Academy Development Group and every literature search conducted has the Academy and LKS branding. This has cemented the now fantastic relationship these two teams have and ensures that the LKS is fully embedded in all quality improvement in the Trust.

Key themes: relationship building, seizing an opportunity, highlighting services and skills, identifying trust priorities

Case Study 4.2 highlights a number of important themes. Most obviously, the need for patience when supporting a trust priority, which in this case was QI. Taking the opportunities offered to the LKS team, however small they seemed, and using those opportunities to advocate for their skills and services at the right moments, eventually led to success. By biding its time, the LKS team not only ensured its own success by being embedded right at the start of the QI process, but it also contributed to the value and success of the QI team.

It is key for knowledge and library specialists to find or make opportunities to meet people within the organisations they serve. There are many ways in which to do this, some of which may include working outside of usual comfort zones, such as manning a stand outside the staff canteen to raise awareness about your service or asking to be invited to meetings that may seem outside of your remit. Identifying promotional activities, such as health awareness days/weeks/months, can be an easy way to identify targeted stakeholder groups as well as highlighting specific services and resources that they will benefit from. It also gives an opportunity to take the work to the stakeholder, for example, taking promotional materials directly to a ward and using the awareness activity as a foot in the door.

Another way in which knowledge and library specialists build relationships within organisations is by attending meetings or joining committees. Many report opportunities arising following attendance at a meeting where they have been able to advocate for the involvement of their services in specific areas of work. For some meetings or committees, such as those related to education, attendance will feel correct given the context of the meeting. Others may feel outside of the usual scope of knowledge and library services, but it is often these sorts of meetings where interesting opportunities arise. Case Study 4.2 is a good example of this. Quality improvement is an area in which many knowledge and library services are now heavily involved, but that was not always the case and it has taken advocacy of skills and services to get to this point.

Once you have identified a committee or meeting where you feel you can support the work being undertaken, for example, a clinical governance committee where you will provide horizon scanning and evidence to underpin effective and robust clinical systems and processes, you may need to advocate for your place in the committee. In relation to the 'principle of social proof', 'one fundamental way that individuals decide what they should do in a situation is to look at what similar people have done' (Cialdini, Wissler and Schweitzer, 2002, 22). Following this principle, in order to prove your place in a committee or meeting, you could supply evidence of similar work being undertaken and the impact it has had, either in your organisation or another. Sometimes, hierarchy can stand in the way of inclusion in meetings, for example, if someone more senior in your structure attends a meeting. In these circumstances, you will need to articulate what you will contribute or gain from attending and how it is different to those already attending. Joining wider groups can also provide you with access to stakeholders you may not network with frequently. This opens up more opportunities and can help you reach across organisations.

Case Study 4.3 below shows how involvement in work beyond the usual knowledge and library services scope can act as an advocacy piece for our professional skills.

Case Study 4.3: Support the refreshing of human resources (HR) policy updates

Team: The King's Fund Library Service

Organisation: The King's Fund

Target group: Human Resources Professionals

How: Following changes to work practices due to the pandemic and the publishing of The King's Fund diversity and inclusion plan for 2022, the library team at The King's Fund was asked to support the refresh and update of HR policies. The service was asked to look for similar HR policies from other organisations to get a sense of what was needed to consider and apply at the Fund. Working with the Head of Diversity and Inclusion to refine what was needed, the team was able to draw best practice from a number of charitable and health sector organisations, as well as other sectors, such as education and local authorities. The findings were presented to the senior management team and ten policies were updated.

Undertaking this work has led to the service being approached for other work related to the diversity and inclusion plans for 2022, including Black History Month and finding people they could potentially collaborate with. Many of the team are involved with internal diversity and inclusion networks and are now actively seeking opportunities to further support this work.

Getting involved in work beyond its usual library and information service expertise has improved the team's visibility within the Fund and has given staff greater awareness of the team's skills and the work it can offer. The King's Fund Library Service say: 'we value the good relationships we have built with key stakeholders. We feel very strongly that relationship building is a core part of the professional skill set.'

Key themes: relationship building, seizing an opportunity, highlighting services and skills, identifying trust priorities

Case Study 4.3 is a good example of extending knowledge and library specialists' skills into a new area and it leading to further opportunities and greater awareness of the service. The involvement in the diversity and inclusion project work spotlights how flexible our professional skills can be in supporting different types of organisational work. Once again, we see the theme of supporting organisational priorities and relationship building. It is essential that knowledge and library specialists advocate for their own professional skills and recognise our authority on evidence, information and knowledge within the organisation. Cialdini, Wissler and Schweitzer (2002, 20–1) argue that people are more easily influenced by those they perceive to be legitimate authorities and who are explicit about their expertise. This can be achieved in a number of ways, including evidencing qualifications, education and professional development. When librarians demonstrate their skills and advocate for the services they offer, they are in fact advocating for the value of the profession (Hicks, 2016, 616), which in turn provides a legacy for knowledge and library services within organisations.

Who should you advocate to?

Before you can begin to build relationships within your organisation and advocate for the role of knowledge and library services in organisational work, you must first have a good knowledge of your stakeholders. Understanding your current users is essential for service planning and delivery and this information can be ascertained through the data collected from service use.

Analysing which staff groups are using your evidence searching services, for example, may tell you which staff groups are routinely using evidence to inform service delivery. Perhaps more importantly, it may also highlight which staff groups are not using knowledge and library services. This will allow you to plan and focus your advocacy efforts.

A successful knowledge and library service will routinely undertake stakeholder mapping exercises to ensure that they are identifying a scale of who is interested in their work versus their level of influence (Quality Improvement East London NHS Foundation Trust, 2019). Using a simple table (see Figure 4.1 below) will let you map your stakeholders and help you plan targeted promotion and marketing. It also ensures that the knowledge and library team are aware of which stakeholders hold the most influence and power.

High power	**Satisfy** These stakeholders will need to be kept satisfied with your services and may need to be regularly reviewed to ensure that they remain in this position.	**Manage** These are your key stakeholders who need to be kept engaged and communicated with regularly.
Low power	**Monitor** This group may be left if you do not have the capacity to support them.	**Inform** This group must be kept aware of services. Their influence may change so you will need to regularly consider their needs and impact.
	Low impact	**High impact**

Figure 4.1 *NHS England, Online Library of Quality Service Improvement and Redesign Tools, 2022*

Utilising user experience (UX) design is another tool to help knowledge and library specialists understand how stakeholders are using their services and how they can improve those services for enhanced use. This is where we begin to think about tailoring services based on the needs of our stakeholders, which may differ from our original intention of service delivery.

Case Study 4.4 below exemplifies a situation where the stakeholder simply wasn't aware of some of the services available for them that had been tailored for their speciality. Instead of continuing to promote those services, the knowledge and library service at North Bristol NHS Trust approached the request by identifying a new way in which they could simplify access.

Case Study 4.4: Mini libraries
Project lead: Sarah Rudd
Trust: North Bristol NHS Trust
Target group: Different specialties, starting with the stroke team
How: The Library and Knowledge team at North Bristol NHS Trust received a request from the stroke department for traditional library support, such as an easily accessible current awareness bulletin and access to an online journal, which was actually already subscribed to by the service. This request came at the same time as a new Trust intranet was launched, which gave the team the ability to create and develop content. The team came up with the idea for 'mini libraries' and they set up three pilot areas with easy access to specialty current awareness bulletins, specific e-resources, journals and links to point-of-care tools. Each mini library is created in consultation with a member of a specialty team to ensure relevance and to support promotion. The mini library sites are built within the specialty intranet area, but are maintained by the library team, which streamlines access and strengthens relationships between the two teams whilst also allowing for fluidity. This project has been a huge success with the number of mini libraries now in double figures.
Key themes: development in technologies, relationship building/building on relationships, 'spreading the word', seizing on an opportunity

---

The creation of mini libraries on the Trust intranet shows the flexibility of service delivery on the part of the knowledge and library services team. The team has developed its own skills to use an alternative platform for the benefit of its stakeholders, putting their needs ahead of how we traditionally assume a stakeholder should access the evidence resources available for them. Once again, we see the theme of relationship building, as well as the principle of social proof (Cialdini, Wissler and Schweitzer, 2002, 22) where the number of mini libraries has grown as other specialties have seen the tailored service that they could also receive.

Many services look beyond the typical service user. NHS England asks that all knowledge and library services have a named board level champion who actively promotes the service (Health Education England, 2022). Broadening the definition of our users is not a recent development, with knowledge and library services supporting decision-making from 'board to ward' (Health Education England, 2021, 7). This allows knowledge and library specialists to support organisational decision-making across all areas, which arguably strengthens our own professional knowledge of healthcare. Case Study 4.5 opposite shows how a relationship built with a new role within the Trust led to involvement in a number of projects, many opportunities for advocacy and high level strategic support from the knowledge and library services team.

Case Study 4.5: Supporting a trust-wide infrastructure for Advanced Clinical Practice

Team/project lead: Epsom and St Helier's University Hospitals NHS Trust Library and Information Service / Potenza Atiogbe

Trust: Epsom and St Helier's University Hospitals NHS Trust

Target group: Advanced Clinical Practitioners (ACPs) and the educators supporting them

Advanced Clinical Practitioners (nursing, midwifery, pharmacists, healthcare scientists and Allied Health Professionals (AHP)) are seen as the future for providing clinical care in local district hospitals where there will be reduced access to the traditional medical workforce. They will be a big part of the clinical workforce for the future.

An investigation of the infrastructure for ACPs at Epsom and St Helier's University Hospitals NHS Trust identified some key gaps, of which 'education and training' was one. This led to the trust applying for and receiving funding for a Lead Educator for Advanced Clinical Practice role. Through an early introduction to the library team and working in the library, a relationship between the library team and the Lead Educator for Advanced Clinical Practice quickly developed and led to numerous opportunities for the service. The support the service offered included technical facilitation of seminars and online learning events. This then meant that the service was given a slot at these events, allowing for promotion of the library service to ACPs, highlighting the specific resources and services on offer to them. For the library team, this led to further involvement in several diverse projects around ACP education, such as ensuring that any policies developed for ACPs were evidence-based, promoting the publication of quality improvement projects related to ACPs, website development, and much more.

Impressively, this has also led to the Library Service Manager being part of the Trust's Strategic Working Group for Advanced Practice and to the Deputy Library Manager co-leading the Research and Evidence-Based Practice Group as part of the ACP and Consultant Practice Level Forum. Future plans include supporting the Trust in creating the proposed Epsom and St Helier's ACP Academy.

Key themes: relationship building, seizing an opportunity, developing technologies, identifying trust priorities

In Case Study 4.5, the initial introduction of the knowledge and library services team to the Lead Educator for Advanced Clinical Practice developed from technical support to leadership opportunities in organisational groups. The team has taken notice of the priorities of the organisations, accepted offered opportunities and advocated for its services and skills to meet newly identified needs. Each healthcare organisation is structured differently and as evidenced above, structures are often shifting or changing. Understanding the structure and nuances within your own organisation, alongside aligning organisational priorities in your strategy and maintaining an awareness of developments in your local health economy will open more possibilities for more groups and people to work with.

Tools of the trade

To ensure that knowledge and library specialists are properly advocating their skills and services, and to enable tailored service delivery, we must ensure that they are given the opportunities to develop these abilities. There are a number of ways in which knowledge and library specialists can learn the soft skills that support advocacy efforts and managers can enable those skills to blossom.

All knowledge and library specialists should be given the opportunity to develop leadership skills. Working inter-professionally with healthcare leaders across vast, complex organisations, knowledge and library specialists must be able to align their work appropriately (Capdarest-Arest and Gray, 2020, 552). This is why it is essential for knowledge and library specialists to have a good understanding of their organisation's strategic priorities and how they tie in to their service. One of the greatest tools a manager can instil in their knowledge and library specialists is an understanding of not only organisational context, but the wider health economy around them. This will allow the knowledge and library specialist to advocate in ways that reflect the needs and priorities of the potential stakeholders who will benefit from them. Having the dual arsenal of leadership skills and context will enable them to speak the language of their audience with authority.

Case Study 4.6: The creation and appointment of a Patient Education Experience Librarian

Team: Sussex Health Knowledge and Libraries
Organisation: University Hospitals Sussex NHS Foundation Trust
Target group: Patients and patient-facing staff
How: Picking up on the increased emphasis on high quality patient information nationally, and following feedback from an inpatient survey, Sussex Health Knowledge and Libraries created a Patient Education Experience Librarian post. Prior to the creation of the post, the Trust had already agreed to build a patient education point within a hospital redevelopment. This meant that the Patient Education Experience Librarian could run the service point, as well as strategically manage the provision of patient information across the hospitals in the Trust and support clinical teams to create high quality patient information.

While creating the post, the team reached out to other services across the country with similar roles to draw on experience. The team also worked with the deputy chief nurse, the patient advice and liaison team and anyone involved with patient experience. This ensured support of the role and gave weight to the role when working with different departments, especially when dealing with patient information that required improvement.

The role has been very successful and has been able to achieve a high profile and impactful service. They have been given the responsibility for chairing the organisation's Carer and Patient Information Group and have established a robust governance process for the production of patient education materials, including creating the Trust's policy for writing patient education materials (which was ratified by the board in 2020). They have created a patient education portal on the Trust's website, began creating video patient information and built closer links with the local public libraries by teaching staff how to identify high quality information online.

Following a merger with another trust, Sussex Health Knowledge and Libraries were asked to lead a working group to align their patient information practices. They are also hoping to increase the capacity of the Patient Education Experience Librarian to further build on the service and ensure equity across the newly merged Trust.

Key themes: Seizing an opportunity, relationship building, identifying trust priorities, using the professional community

Identifying alternative skills within a team to support new endeavours can often be key to successful projects. Facilitation skills can be learnt by library and knowledge specialists through professional development opportunities, but is often naturally part of a librarian's skill set. For activities related to knowledge mobilisation for example, facilitation skills are intrinsic to the offer. Successful knowledge and library service teams are open to exploring and extending their skills and will often take advantage of professional development opportunities to develop their soft skills alongside traditional librarian skills, as seen in CILIP's PKSB. Managers should be using the PKSB during annual reviews and skills mapping exercises to understand skills gaps, working with and encouraging their team members to grow those skills and therefore their confidence. Elevator pitches are an easy way to prepare for situations in which a knowledge and library specialist may find themselves advocating. By preparing the main point of promotion, the knowledge and library specialist can feel confident in their knowledge, what they want to get across and know that they are being succinct. It will allow them to build on conversations without worrying that they have missed any key points. Elevator pitches practice is often included within leadership programmes and has recently been included in the curriculum of bespoke advocacy and influencing training commissioned by HEE for the newly created Primary Care Knowledge Specialist role.

Throughout this chapter, the discussion has placed the onus on knowledge and library specialists advocating for their services. However, library champions can be an important tool, not just in helping you to advocate, but also acting as an advocate to other staff within the organisation. Library champions can also identify new opportunities for the involvement of services. Knowledge and library services teams should spend time identifying and building library champions within their organisations to support their endeavours and involvement in organisational projects. Champions do not have to be formal, they just need to understand the relevance of the knowledge and library service to their colleagues so that word of mouth promotion grows.

Resilience is also a key skill for knowledge and library specialists, particularly within healthcare. Knowledge and library specialists who are putting themselves out there and advocating for their services in situations that they might not usually find themselves in, need to be equipped with resilience and coping skills. There will be times when they are told no, are asked why they are at a meeting or are rejected from being involved in a project. This can be a deeply uncomfortable experience. Knowledge and library teams can support each other in building resilience and coping skills by debriefing each other following advocacy efforts. Not only will this support colleagues who feel let down, but it can also act as a learning opportunity for everyone in the team. This will prevent colleagues becoming disheartened and hopefully ensure that they feel confident enough to seek future opportunities.

Challenges

Alongside the positives, advocacy can come with challenges. Advocacy often acts as its own form of marketing and promotion. Once a successful project has bedded in, other stakeholder groups are able to see how it could benefit them. This can sometimes mean that knowledge and library services teams are flooded with requests and so must consider the capacity and strengths of the team. Although this increased demand can be used to argue for increasing team capacity or filling skills gaps, this may be difficult where organisations are facing cost savings. There may be instances where tough decisions about where to focus efforts are made and services have to say 'no' or stagger their engagement opportunities.

Librarians in healthcare may also come across conflicts of interest; for example, within the NHS, those interests set out by the organisation they serve and the delivery expected by HEE, the stewards of knowledge and library services in the NHS in England. The ambitions set out in HEE's Knowledge for Healthcare (2021) determine the strategic direction for health knowledge and library services, which may not seem in line with the strategic priorities set out by host organisations. The challenge that knowledge and library services face is translating what we can offer professionally, as set out in Knowledge for Healthcare, to support the priorities of the organisation. Some organisations have a lack of understanding about the vast skills on offer from knowledge and library specialists and instead focus on traditional library services or the space. It is the responsibility of the librarian to make those translations to see how those seeming conflicts actually work together to align with the priorities of the organisation and Knowledge for Healthcare.

Conclusion

Advocacy of knowledge and library services and knowledge and library specialists, our skills and what we have to offer is vital:

- All library staff have an essential role to play in advocating and they must be armed with the skills and knowledge to do so.
- High quality knowledge and library teams are able to vocalise how their unique skill sets and resources can enhance projects or developments happening within health organisations.
- They regularly assess their stakeholders and map their needs to service provision and plan for service development in line with their advocacy effort.
- There is a good understanding throughout the team of the priorities of their organisation, developments nationally and in the local health economy.
- Flexibility is evident in the delivery of services based on the needs of their stakeholders.

> Be open to try something new. Believe that you don't have to do anything extra. We had the skills, resources and the willingness and they were matched with the needs of the ACPs and our profession was viewed as an equal partner.
> (Potenza Atiogbe, from Case Study 4.5 above)

As you take your advocacy forward, here are three things to reflect on:

1 Have you considered the importance of advocacy in knowledge and library services?

2 Using CILIP's PKSB, how would you rate your current advocacy skills?
3 What professional development could you undertake to enhance your advocacy skills?

References

Capdarest-Arest, N. and Gray, J. M. (2020) Health Sciences Library Leadership Skills in an Interprofessional Landscape: A Review And Textual Analysis, *Journal of the Medical Library Association*, **108** (4), 547–55.

Cialdini, R. B., Wissler, R. L. and Schweitzer, N. J. (2002) The Science of Influence, *Dispute Resolution Magazine*, **9**, 20–2.

CILIP (2022) *Professional Knowledge and Skills Base, Section 11, Generic Skills – Leadership, Advocacy, Influencing and Personal Effectiveness.* https://pksb.cilip.org.uk/section/generic-skills/leadership-advocacy-influencing-and-personal-effectiveness.

Health Education England (2021) *Knowledge for Healthcare: Mobilising Evidence; Sharing Knowledge; Improving Outcomes. A Strategic Framework for NHS Knowledge and Library Services 2021–2026.* www.hee.nhs.uk/our-work/knowledge-for-healthcare.

Health Education England Knowledge and Library Services (2022) *Plan on a Page.* https://library.hee.nhs.uk/learning-academy/learning-zone/plan-on-a-page.

Hicks, D. (2016) Advocating for Librarianship: The Discourses of Advocacy and Service in the Professional Identity of Librarians, *Library Trends*, **64** (3), 615–40.

NHS England (2022) *Online Library of Quality, Service Improvement and Redesign Tools: Stakeholder Analysis.* www.england.nhs.uk/wp-content/uploads/2022/02/qsir-stakeholder-analysis.pdf.

Quality Improvement East London NHS Foundation Trust (2019) *Resources – Stakeholder Mapping Tool.* https://qi.elft.nhs.uk/wp-content/uploads/2019/11/2.-Stakeholder-Mapping-Tool.pptx.pdf.

Secker, J. and Walton, G. (2015) *UK Information Literacy Advocacy: Reaching Out Beyond the Tower.* European Conference on Information Literacy (ECIL), Tallinn, Estonia.

UCL (2022) *Information Studies Postgraduate Study.* www.ucl.ac.uk/module-catalogue/modules/managing-information-organisations/INST0021.

Further reading

Jaeger, P., Zerhusen, E., Gorham, U., Hill, R. F. and Greene Taylor, N. (2017) Waking Up to Advocacy in a New Political Reality for Libraries, *The Library Quarterly*, **87** (4), 350–68.

5

Mobilising Evidence and Knowledge

Emily Hopkins and Katie Nicholas

Introduction and strategic context

Regarding mobilising evidence and knowledge, Knowledge for Healthcare states:

> … healthcare is a knowledge industry. Decisions are not made in isolation but must take account of individual and organisational knowledge as well as the best available evidence. NHS knowledge specialists enable decision makers to take account of this full continuum. They also nurture a learning culture which is critical to transformation, efficiency and innovation within the NHS.
>
> (Health Education England, 2021)

This opens up the role of knowledge and library specialists to become active partners, along with clinical and managerial colleagues, in the use of evidence and knowledge by healthcare organisations. It allows them to contribute by not only providing easy access to published information and evidence, but also to play a key part in making it useful and usable and facilitating the better capture and use of knowledge gained in the organisation.

As Knowledge for Healthcare and the National Institute for Health Research acknowledge:

> … evidence does not speak for itself but needs to be mobilised at the right time, and through the right people, to make a difference in decision making.
>
> (National Institute for Health Research, 2013)

While evidence-based practice is seen as the gold standard in healthcare organisations and people are willing in principle to use evidence in their decision-making, the practical challenges of doing so are where the skills of knowledge specialists can make a difference.

The role of mobilising evidence and knowledge requires skills in the use of information, as well as skills in using the technology to harness it. It involves working as an embedded part of teams, including clinical, managerial, policy development and project teams. As well as honing search skills to find the right information, knowledge specialists working in this space find themselves called upon to summarise and present the evidence in a digestible format to help take the 'heavy lifting' out of getting the evidence into practice (Economics by Design, 2020).

Although this chapter does not cover the concept of mobilising computable biomedical knowledge, it is worth noting that this too is an area of increasing interest where knowledge specialists' skills are relevant and there are likely to be developments here in the future. Technical and information skills, such as semantic web standards and knowledge of taxonomy and metadata, are being called upon to help in organising individual, actionable units of knowledge. This can include supplying key clinical guideline recommendations within patient record systems, ensuring clinicians always see the most up to date prescribing or other guidance at the point of care. For further exploration in the area of mobilising computable biomedical knowledge, the Topol Review (NHS, 2019) gives an insight into the digital future of the health sector and the Faculty of Clinical Informatics (2023) in particular is leading developments in this area.

Facilitation is also a key skill, with knowledge specialists increasingly being involved in facilitating knowledge mobilisation tools, explained in detail later in this chapter, for teams seeking to capture and share their knowledge and learning. Not only are knowledge specialists often essential to the effective facilitation of these tools, but they also act as champions, helping drive an organisational culture that is positive about sharing knowledge, seeking evidence and learning from innovations and new ideas.

While much of this may seem removed from the traditional librarian role, it also builds on information skills and understanding the knowledge needs of the teams the knowledge specialist is working with, transitioning from providing access to the evidence to becoming a collaborator in putting it into practice. Knowledge specialists increasingly have a reputation as trusted partners for knowledge and evidence, delivering the Knowledge for Healthcare aim that:

> Healthcare organisations, services and systems effectively mobilise evidence, learning, knowledge and 'know how' to enable evidence-based policy and practice.
>
> (Health Education England, 2021)

Defining mobilising evidence and knowledge

Terminology and definitions can often be seen as jargon and a barrier to knowledge specialists feeling confident that they have the right knowledge and skills to work in this area. Definitions can vary across sectors too, with knowledge management having its origins in commercial and business sectors rather than health, and in many cases focusing on the tacit knowledge of employees, perhaps with less of an emphasis on research evidence. In healthcare, the emphasis is often on both evidence and knowledge as they are complementary to each other in a healthcare setting.

It often helps to define some broad terms used in this area and the terms used in this chapter. There is clearly some overlap and these terms are not mutually exclusive – managing knowledge also involves mobilising it for example – and knowledge management experts, particularly from other sectors, may disagree over some details, such as whether once captured, knowledge becomes information! However, below are some broad, pragmatic definitions used in the health sector that give an overall picture of the priorities in this area and what is meant by mobilising evidence and knowledge:

- **Evidence**: The available published literature or research on a topic.
- **Evidence-based practice**: The principle of ensuring that healthcare and management decision-making are based on evidence, but also informed by the knowledge of the experts involved.
- **Knowledge**: Awareness, information, facts and understanding gathered through education and experience. It may already be captured in recorded form and turned into knowledge assets, or exist as tacit knowledge and 'know-how', held in people's heads and captured and shared through the knowledge mobilisation techniques described below.
- **Knowledge management**: The process of creating, sharing, managing and applying knowledge by an organisation, including soft intelligence held by individuals, and relevant evidence.
- **Knowledge mobilisation**: Enabling an organisation to use its knowledge as an asset for decision-making and service improvement.
- **Knowledge translation**: The process of putting knowledge into action, using knowledge to inform decisions in healthcare policy and practice. A dynamic and iterative process that includes the synthesis, dissemination, exchange and application of knowledge derived from research.

Typical service overview: what does mobilising evidence and knowledge look like in the health sector? How does it fit with library services?

As is likely already apparent through this book, there is no single type of knowledge and library service or team structure in the health sector. The team composition varies according to organisational size, design and needs.

It is worth considering the range and variety of healthcare organisations and types of knowledge, evidence and information they will use and how best to mobilise it. Healthcare providers, such as GP surgeries and hospitals, will need easy and timely access to up-to-date clinical evidence at the point of care, to inform decisions about individual patients, including information for prescribing medicines, referral pathways and other treatment options. Often information and evidence will be presented in easily digestible formats through point of care tools for quick and easy access. Clinical staff will also need easy access to new research to keep up to date with the evolving evidence in their specialty area and to ensure they always provide the best care for their patients.

Other healthcare organisations are concerned with planning and design of healthcare services. In England, this includes Integrated Care Systems planning services for the region they serve and national bodies setting policy and guidance for the whole country. NHS England leads policy development and commissioning for healthcare services in England and, through its Workforce Training and Education Directorate (formerly known as Health Education England), plans and trains the healthcare workforce. NICE leads development of clinical guidance and quality standards. Such organisations will often require a range of evidence and knowledge throughout project and policy development cycles, understanding the impact of clinical research on the structure and delivery of healthcare services and implications for training staff. Equivalent bodies and activities of course exist in the rest of the UK.

When it comes to mobilising evidence and knowledge, at one end of the spectrum, what may be considered traditional health library services often focus on providing the evidence through easy access to resources, such as books and journals, and carrying out literature searches, including by embedded clinical librarian and knowledge specialist roles. These services are often branching out by building on their literature searching services, producing evidence summaries and syntheses to help make the evidence more easily usable. A further step may involve knowledge specialists running or assisting with knowledge mobilisation tools and techniques, for example, facilitating an after action review following a change introduced by a team to their processes and procedures.

At the more embedded knowledge management end of the spectrum, often in regional and national organisations that provide oversight and leadership of healthcare services, it is perhaps more obvious to see how knowledge management practices can be embedded within policy development and project management cycles. The authors' own team, the Knowledge Management Service in NHS England's Workforce Training and Education Directorate, provides a comprehensive range of knowledge management activities. Knowledge specialists are aligned to and embedded within teams as needed to provide different services and activities as required. They can work alongside colleagues at different points throughout a project to provide advice and input on knowledge management processes as needed. Having aligned knowledge management support in this way helps teams assess and improve their own knowledge management practices and ensure their work is well evidenced and their knowledge is captured. The knowledge specialists can guide the team in question through the Self-Assessment Tool (described below) to help assess their current practices and where they would like to improve. They can then recommend tools and techniques from the knowledge mobilisation framework, as well as provide literature searching and evidence summaries as required throughout the project.

An example area of work for an NHS England Workforce, Training and Education team could be a project to develop policies and training approaches for new healthcare roles or innovations in healthcare education delivery, such as using virtual reality (VR) to help deliver training to healthcare students and staff. The knowledge specialist will carry out searches to scope the evidence base from the UK and internationally, looking for good practice, reports and policies, as well as primary research. They may also set up current awareness alerts to keep people up to date with new publications. They can also advise on and even facilitate a tool, such as an after action review or retrospect, to capture the learning as the project is implemented, or a peer assist to learn from a similar team elsewhere. This could include the project team members, as well as participants from pilot sites adopting the new roles or testing the VR technology, to capture their learning for future use. Involvement at multiple stages of the project helps the knowledge specialist to act as a trusted partner and tailor the advice and services provided. This often includes offering advice proactively or working to link teams together to encourage knowledge sharing and the development of communities of practice.

NHS Knowledge Mobilisation Framework

The NHS Knowledge Mobilisation Framework (Health Education England Knowledge and Library Services, 2021a) is a set of techniques designed for use in settings across the NHS. It is designed to be flexible and provides a selection of tools to choose from as appropriate, rather than needing to use the whole framework. The framework is organised into three areas (Learning Before, Learning During, Learning After), encouraging the use of evidence and the sharing and capturing of knowledge at all stages of a project or piece of work.

Table 5.1 *NHS Knowledge Mobilisation Framework*

Learning Before	Learning During	Learning After
Self-Assessment Tool Peer Assist Before Action Review Appreciative Inquiry	After Action Reviews Knowledge Café Randomised Coffee Trials Communities of Practice Action Learning Sets Knowledge Assets Fishbowl	Knowledge Harvesting Retrospect

These stages, as well as the tools and techniques of the framework, are described in more detail below.

Learning Before

The techniques included in the Learning Before section are designed to help teams assess their use of knowledge and identify opportunities to make better use of knowledge as they set out on a new piece of work. They encourage teams to think about others who have done something similar and consider if there is learning that can be harnessed or good practice that can be replicated. Techniques support taking time to consider what the team is setting out to achieve, learning from the experience of themselves and others, and understanding what success might look like, as well as offering space to generate ideas and stimulate innovation.

Learning During

The techniques included in the Learning During section support continuous learning and reflection throughout the project or piece of work. This includes facilitating conversations amongst individuals so they can share ideas and connecting people to each other to help them solve problems and build communities. The tools also offer ways to package the knowledge captured in accessible and usable formats, so others can benefit from the learning.

Learning After

This assists teams in capturing learning at the end stages of a project. It includes structured approaches to capturing experience as a project team disbands or if someone is leaving. It also offers opportunities to reflect on whether project objectives were achieved; to highlight successes and consider how they could be repeated; and to acknowledge failures and consider how they could be avoided in future. These techniques provide the opportunity to reflect on how the project could have been improved so learning can be shared, mistakes avoided in future and good practice replicated.

A collection of e-learning modules (eLearning for Healthcare, 2018) and a set of postcards (Health Education England Knowledge and Library Services, 2021a) are also available to introduce the framework and techniques. These can be used to reflect and plan activities as a team, as prompts to facilitate learning activities and to promote organisational learning and knowledge sharing.

Tools, techniques and terminology

Knowledge management terminology can be intimidating. Table 5.2 below outlines some key techniques and associated terminology, with plain language definitions and examples of how they might be applied to real-world scenarios.

Table 5.2 *Knowledge management terminology – tools and techniques*

Self-Assessment Tool	**A simple framework to quickly assess how the team or** organisation can make better use of knowledge as an asset and identify opportunities to develop and learn. *When might this be used?* In team planning, to identify knowledge and evidence needs and areas for development.
Peer Assist	A structured, facilitated meeting or workshop where peers are invited from other teams or organisations to provide their experience, insights and knowledge to a team who have requested help. *When might this be used?* At the start of a project, consider reaching out to colleagues with relevant experience from other departments or sectors.
Before Action Review	Helps the team state their intention (task, purpose and end-state) just before commencing the project, project stage or a piece of work. It also adds the discipline of predicting challenges and risks and, most importantly, drawing lessons learned from past experiences. *When might this be used?* At the start of a big project or piece of work, schedule a conversation as a project team to map out objectives and discuss potential challenges.
Appreciative Inquiry	A different way to see and be in the world, to learn and build on what teams already do well rather than focusing upon problems. Appreciative Inquiry can generate ideas, energise changes and stimulate innovation on a large scale. It uses five key questions looking at Definition, Discovery, Dream, Design and Delivery. *When might this be used?* Use this in an organisation to generate new ideas with colleagues and spark innovation.

Continued

Table 5.2 *Continued*

After Action Review	A short, structured meeting held immediately after a short-term activity, such as a task within a project; for example, a training session, a go live day or an engagement meeting. Usually facilitated by one of the team members. All who were involved in the 'action' should participate. *When might this be used?* At the end of the first phase of a project, check in with the project team to assess progress and share learning that can inform the next project phase.
Knowledge Café	A conversational technique consisting of small tables of conversational groups, focusing on an overall question or topic. Participants swap tables every 15 minutes to begin a new conversation, meet new people, get a fresh perspective on the topic and to encourage people to learn from each other. The value is in the conversation itself and the learning that everyone takes away. *When might this be used?* Use as part of an event to help attendees come together and discuss a hot topic or problem and potential solutions.
Randomised Coffee Trials	Enables people to meet and connect with one another at random, giving them time to talk about whatever they wish, perhaps over a cup of coffee. They help build relationships, improve communication and encourage collaboration and the sharing of knowledge and ideas. *When might this be used?* As part of an induction programme, arrange chats for new starters to help them meet colleagues from other teams.
Communities of Practice	A group of individuals who come together to share ideas, develop expertise and solve problems around a topic of interest. They can be made up of people across the NHS and beyond, so that knowledge is shared and used widely. *When might this be used?* Identify individuals and bring them together as a group to discuss a shared issue or areas of expertise.
Action Learning Sets	A supportive environment, enabling small groups to meet regularly to discuss, reflect and find solutions to work-related issues or to develop skills in a common area of interest. This tool is especially geared to learning and personal development. *When might this be used?* As a professional development tool – meet with other people from a course to coach one another.

Continued

Table 5.2 *Continued*

Knowledge Assets	Knowledge and experience, captured and packaged in one place to be of maximum use to people who could benefit from that learning in the future. They may contain lessons learned, case histories, key contacts and best practice. *When might this be used?* As the project progresses, write case studies detailing the learning, mistakes and successes and make them available for others to read.
Fishbowl	A conversational technique for debating hot topics or sharing ideas and knowledge from a variety of perspectives. All participants sit in a circle, around three or four chairs in an inner circle that are occupied by those speaking. Participants can join and leave the inner circle as required, with the facilitator ensuring people have an opportunity to speak and that the Fishbowl is inclusive. *When might this be used?* As an alternative panel in a conference agenda, allowing a dynamic conversation to develop with attendees.
Knowledge Harvesting	A structured approach to help an organisation understand and record the knowledge and experience of people, often before they leave or move roles. *When might this be used?* If a member of staff is leaving the project team or organisation, arrange a facilitated conversation with them to capture their unique knowledge and expertise.
Retrospect	A structured facilitated meeting or workshop at the end of a project (or a major project stage) to capture the knowledge before the team disbands. *When might this be used?* After a project has ended, bring the project team together to discuss the successes and achievements. Record key learning for the future and make it available to other teams.
Evidence Summary and Synthesis	The results of a literature search presented as a summarised or synthesised report. This may pull out key themes or highlight must-read pieces of evidence. This includes searching peer reviewed journal literature, reports or policy documents and other literature relevant to the topic. A summary will usually provide a high level synopsis of key themes as a guide to the evidence, whereas a synthesis is more detailed, often including formal critical appraisal of the evidence it cites and drawing conclusions. *When might this be used?* As part of a project plan, consider the evidence at the early stages, look at literature to inform the business case or decision-making. A summary or synthesis will help get team members and stakeholders familiar with the evidence quickly, even if they don't have the time or expertise to read every published paper in depth.

Continued

Table 5.2 *Continued*

Current Awareness and Horizon Scanning	The distribution to subscribers of information about the latest news, publications and research, a core offering of many knowledge and library services. Usually offered as a regular e-mail bulletin.
	When might this be used? During the piece of work, consider setting up some alerts or signing up to some relevant bulletins to stay up to date with newly published research that may inform the project as it develops.

Mobilising evidence in practice

The evidence does not speak for itself, but when talking about 'mobilising evidence', what does that mean in practice? How does it differ from providing access to evidence and knowledge through library services or carrying out literature searches?

Mobilising evidence is indeed an extension of those familiar services, but with an emphasis on presenting the evidence in such a way as to make it more easily navigable and actionable. Examples would include: providing a summary of the evidence identified through a literature search to highlight key points and themes; assisting the reader in finding the actionable recommendations quickly and easily, highlighting aspects such as the country or sector to help the reader assess relevance; or grouping articles by theme and providing a short narrative summary or introduction to explain the overall picture of the evidence base and any gaps or areas where evidence is lacking.

Of course, this is easier for the knowledge specialist to do for less technical topics, such as management reports and policy documents. Building up a sound understanding of these topics to assist with producing summaries is a key part of the knowledge specialist's role. For more advanced areas of work, however, this may progress to working with teams to provide structured critical appraisal and develop a synthesis of the evidence, creating what is effectively a new piece of evidence in its own right. Skills in teaching critical appraisal tools and processes are key here and complement those of colleagues with subject matter expertise. The knowledge specialist can help subject matter experts assess the quality of information and determine its quality, weight and relevance to the topic in hand and what needs to be taken on board.

Clearly, for clinical information or anything where medical or technical expertise is required, the knowledge specialist alone would not be expected to have the expertise to summarise or synthesise such information. They will, however, find themselves working in conjunction with colleagues with clinical or other subject matter expertise to produce such summaries and syntheses. Here, the key skills of the knowledge specialist are again in the presentation and accessibility of information, along with understanding how users search and the barriers that users can face. This gives an insight into how to present information in an accessible and actionable format, rather than recommendations buried in long article text, and using the principles of knowledge translation to ensure the focus is on presenting the evidence in an actionable format – focusing on what the reader or recipient needs to do to put it into practice.

Mobilising knowledge in practice

As described above, organisational knowledge can take a variety of formats, although it is most often held in people's heads – either built up through experience or relatively new learning acquired through a project or piece of work. In some senses, mobilising knowledge is the opposite problem to mobilising evidence. While evidence is usually well indexed and relatively easy to find with the right access to databases, finding the people with the right knowledge can often rely more on luck and attempting to capture their knowledge in a useful, structured format can take considerable effort. Also, capturing and storing knowledge is only useful if there is someone, or there is likely to be someone in the future, to make use of it. Enabling conversations and peer-to-peer learning can often be as effective and enable immediate action.

Again, the knowledge specialist's role here is to use their skills to understand colleagues' needs and help them elicit the right knowledge through questions and discussion, capturing the right notes, where appropriate, to ensure key new knowledge is recorded either for participants to action immediately or to produce a knowledge asset so that the knowledge is recorded and not lost. Group facilitation is a key skill and being able to manage a group in person and online, encouraging equal participation and a productive discussion, is vital. Knowledge specialists often find themselves in a role as a neutral third party to help bring that fresh perspective to discussions and give the team the time and space to reflect and share their learning and knowledge, using an appropriate tool from the knowledge mobilisation framework.

A team or organisation at a higher level of maturity with knowledge mobilisation will not always need the knowledge specialist to act as facilitator; project teams who are well practiced may automatically build in an after action review at every project stage and self-facilitate this. In some organisations, this may also be a role undertaken by functions such as organisational development or learning and development teams.

Knowledge specialists have a unique perspective as they are skilled in understanding and facilitating knowledge mobilisation activities and evidence mobilisation. Working with colleagues to help them understand the power of both evidence and knowledge – and using them in combination to best effect – helps knowledge specialists play a key part in ensuring their organisations are well informed and are taking action based on the best available evidence combined with relevant knowledge.

The knowledge mobilisation self-assessment tool

Mobilising evidence and knowledge takes a variety of forms and serves a variety of purposes. The knowledge specialist and the services they provide are a key part of this. However, it also requires teams and organisations to be active participants and play their part in achieving success. An organisational culture of willingness to share knowledge and seek out evidence, with senior leaders, in particular, appreciating the value of knowledge as an asset, is fundamental to success. The role of the knowledge specialist is one of champion and change agent, but organisations must also actively participate and embed knowledge mobilisation practices throughout its processes. Knowledge specialists can provide expert facilitation, but many of the knowledge mobilisation tools can also be self-facilitated by teams.

The knowledge mobilisation self-assessment tool (Health Education England Knowledge and Library Services, 2021b) is a maturity model developed by Knowledge for Healthcare, to help organisations assess their current level of maturity in this area and identify where they want to make improvements. This may be individual teams within the organisation or a board taking an organisation-wide view to spread good practice and improve the overall maturity beyond pockets of good practice.

Knowledge specialists can use this tool to facilitate a conversation with a team or department to help them understand their current practices and make recommendations for improvement. This may be simple changes the team can adopt themselves or helping them understand how to make better use of the knowledge and library service to support their knowledge management practices.

Measuring impact

Evaluating and measuring the quality and impact of knowledge and library services is of course vital, as discussed in Chapter 10. Measuring the impact of knowledge and evidence mobilisation activities is no exception. While the tools for measuring impact of evidence services are well established, tools to measure the impact of knowledge mobilisation tools and activities are still at a relatively early stage of development at the time of writing. Through Knowledge for Healthcare, the existing impact tools are being developed to account for knowledge mobilisation and the impacts this may have, plus how it may be similar to, and differ from, evidence mobilisation. Further development of tools and approaches to look at the impact from an individual, team, organisation and health system level are also in progress, acknowledging the fact that this is not a single transaction. Knowledge is captured, used and shared throughout organisations and systems in a constantly evolving manner.

This of course makes monitoring impact tricky as the outcomes of a particular knowledge mobilisation activity may not be seen immediately and can be more of a chain reaction of sharing knowledge and building relationships within and across teams. For example, an after action review can capture useful immediate knowledge and learning from a project and then also foster a deeper trust within the team concerned, helping discover knowledge about which colleagues can be drawn upon later and revealing the 'go to' people on particular topics.

As standardised tools become available across NHS knowledge and library services, it will become easier and more commonplace to evaluate the use of knowledge mobilisation tools and understand the overall impact knowledge management activities have on organisations, particularly when combined with the maturity assessment offered by the self-assessment tool. The overall principle of better understanding the value of evidence and knowledge and the difference made by making this easily accessible, useful and actionable is important to ensure services in this area make a real contribution to decision-making around healthcare services and, ultimately, patient care.

Case studies: examples of evidence and knowledge mobilisation

As outlined earlier in this chapter, services and activities can vary depending on the organisation and environment. Below are some examples of real-life activities happening in different types of healthcare settings in the NHS in England.

Case Study 5.1: Building a repository of ambulance service research – capturing knowledge and evidence produced by ambulance staff

Team/project lead: Matt Holland, Library Manager at Library and Knowledge Service for NHS Ambulance Services in England

Trust: North West Ambulance Service / NHS Ambulance Services in England

The Library and Knowledge Service for NHS Ambulance Services in England was tasked with delivering a repository solution for ambulance services in England. They purchased OpenRepository software and created Amber – the home of ambulance service research. Working with Manchester University NHS Trust Library, over 1,300 items have been added, many of which are not found on major databases. Amber is integrated into the National Ambulance Research Steering Group (NARSG) website to showcase research and is a key resource for students and researchers. It provides a focus for ambulance service and paramedic research where there was previously none. Its development coincides with the emergence of these topics as distinct areas of research.

Case Study 5.2: Randomised Coffee Trials at a large mental health and disability NHS trust – connecting staff to help share learning

Team/project lead: Suzanne Wilson, Head of Library and Knowledge Services
Trust: Cumbria, Northumberland, Tyne and Wear NHS Foundation Trust
The team recognised the challenges of staying connected with colleagues after the rise of home working during the pandemic. The 'corridor conversations' and serendipitous exchanges of experience that contribute to shared learning were increasingly difficult. The team encouraged staff to sign up to be randomly paired with another member of staff to have a conversation. A welcome email is sent inviting people to meet with their pair using Microsoft Teams. Participants report it helps them make valuable new connections and learn about other teams in the organisation.

Case Study 5.3: Knowledge Cafés to support health and wellbeing conversations in an acute and community NHS trust

Team/project lead: Susan Smith, Library Manager at Joint Education and Training (JET) Library
Trust: Mid Cheshire Hospitals NHS Foundation Trust
The library team at Mid Cheshire Hospitals NHS Foundation Trust run facilitated Knowledge Cafés for Trust and Clinical Commissioning Group (CCG) staff in the region. The Cafés cover topics of growing interest and importance that previously have had less focus and awareness, although staff are likely to have experience to share. This includes health and wellbeing, the menopause and sustainability.

Case Study 5.4: Facilitation skills and embedded working in an acute and community NHS trust

Team/project lead: Laura Wilkes, Knowledge and Library Services Manager

Trust: West Suffolk NHS Trust
The Knowledge and Library Service Manager at West Suffolk NHS Trust helped facilitate a series of workshops in the Trust that led to an embedded role supporting a flexible working programme and facilitating further workshops with managers. Following on from this project, they are now working with the Quality Improvement team to collate themes and identify further improvement projects.

Case Study 5.5: A Knowledge Management team in a national NHS body

Team/project lead: Emily Hopkins, Knowledge Management Service Lead
Organisation: NHS England Workforce, Training and Education Directorate
The authors' own team, the Knowledge Management Service at NHS England Workforce Training and Education (formerly known as Health Education England), facilitates after action reviews and retrospects with teams to capture learning, for example when developing new training programmes for healthcare staff. They are embedded in major review teams, in areas such as the impact of new technology on nursing and midwifery training, compiling evidence summaries that inform the review as it progresses. They also assist teams to produce case studies on workforce and education topics for the eWIN collection on the NHS Learning Hub. These include key learning points for anyone seeking to undertake a similar project.

See also Chapter 11 for an example of after action reviews for reflective practice.

Reflective exercise

Having read the chapter, you may be wondering what it is really like working to mobilise evidence and knowledge. What sort of things would you be involved in? What challenges might you need to tackle and how would you apply your skills? The following scenario is fictionalised, but is based on fairly common, real scenarios that knowledge specialists face. It gives you the chance to put yourself in the shoes of a knowledge specialist working in this area.

Read through the scenario and think about techniques and expertise you could use to support the team in their use of knowledge and evidence at all stages of their project.

You are a knowledge specialist in a knowledge and library service team in a large hospital.
The Paediatrics (children's) ward team have been working on a project to improve bedside handover protocol. This is a procedure that all staff follow when transferring from one shift to another to update the incoming shift on the patient's current condition. Initially, the team wanted to review existing evidence on handover protocols and managing medication mistakes and learn if there was any new evidence here. *Prompt: How might you support the team in engaging with existing evidence?*
As a result of their project, the team implemented a small change that vastly improved the process and eliminated medication mistakes completely. The patients and their parents and carers are also much happier as it gives them more opportunity to ask questions about their treatment and to be introduced to their new nursing team, which they find reassuring. Overall, it has been a great success. *Prompt: What techniques might you use to help the team reflect on their progress and make sure learning isn't forgotten now the new protocol is business as usual?*
You know that the team in the Oncology (cancer) ward are also looking at updating their protocols around their own handover process. *Prompt: How might you support teams to learn from colleagues?*
The hospital has many different departments who haven't reviewed their protocols recently either, although due to other priorities it's unlikely that they'll want to do this very soon. *Prompt: How might you share the learning across the organisation?*

Figure 5.1 *Scenario: bedside handover in a hospital setting*

The aim was for you to reflect on how and when the techniques can be applied and which might be most appropriate for a given situation. There are no specific right answers, however, below are some suggestions of techniques you might consider.

The team wanted to review existing evidence – the knowledge and library service could conduct a literature search, summarise the evidence and make the key points easy to locate so the team can digest the latest research and apply it. In order to help the team stay up to date with evidence throughout their project, you might also set up alerts to keep the team informed about the latest publications so they don't miss emerging research published after they have started their project.

During the project you could facilitate after action reviews with the team so that they can check in and share learning as they reach the end of a phase. To support the team's reflection on their learning at the end of the project, you could facilitate a retrospect – a longer, more detailed look back at the whole project that will help them elicit their key learning and capture this as a report or knowledge asset.

As you know the Oncology ward also want to update their protocols, you could facilitate a Peer Assist linking them with the Paediatrics team so they can ask questions and share their learning.

Other departments may want to learn from good practice when they look to update their protocols in the future. You could work with the Paediatrics team to create a case study highlighting their work, including key learning, and make it available for colleagues in the rest of the organisation to read. Not only does this help them celebrate their success, it also highlights learning and innovation in the organisation.

The purpose of this exercise was to think about how you might help mobilise evidence and knowledge to solve a practical problem or make a positive difference to practice in a healthcare setting.

The future

This area, like many others in the world of health information, is constantly evolving, with ongoing developments growing the possibilities for knowledge specialist roles and useful applications of key knowledge specialist skills. Predicting the future may run the risk of over-optimism; however, the growth so far and the relevance to improving evidence-based practice suggests a strong foundation on which knowledge specialists can build.

This chapter has not covered the vast possibilities of mobilising computable biomedical knowledge. This is an area of increasing demand that will need the skills not only of expert clinicians and technical staff but, increasingly, those of information professionals and knowledge specialists. These skills will bridge the gap between the technical systems and tools and the information skills needed to make them most useful. Skills such as taxonomy, metadata and semantic web standards are key to making the vast data sets useful, relevant and available to the right people at the right time.

Acting as embedded knowledge specialists within teams, using tools such as the self-assessment tool described in this chapter and impact measurement tools, will also become more commonplace as healthcare organisations and teams develop their maturity in this area. The role of the knowledge specialist will be in ever-increasing demand, helping organisations understand their knowledge needs and providing expert facilitation to make best use of knowledge and evidence.

Conclusion

Mobilising evidence and knowledge is an area of growing importance and relevance. It is also one that is satisfying to work in. Knowledge specialists working in this area are likely to be embedded within wider teams and therefore see the knowledge and evidence they provide being put into use immediately, having a positive influence on decision-making and organisational effectiveness. Core information skills, such as searching and critical appraisal, are obviously key, but this area also provides the opportunity to develop facilitation skills and work as part of multi-disciplinary teams with a wide variety of work.

The future possibilities are ever-expanding. Technology offers some solutions, but the skills of knowledge specialists will always be needed to ensure knowledge and evidence are captured as needed, quality and relevance are determined, and that they are useful and actionable. And, above all, to ensure organisations have the right approach and an appetite for seeking and sharing knowledge and evidence.

References

Economics by Design (2020) *NHS Funded Library and Knowledge Services in England – Value Proposition: The Gift of Time*. www.hee.nhs.uk/our-work/library-knowledge-services/value-proposition-gift-time.

eLearning for Healthcare (2018) *Knowledge Mobilisation Framework*. www.e-lfh.org.uk/programmes/knowledge-mobilisation-framework.

Faculty of Clinical Informatics (2023) *UK Activity on Mobilising Computable Biomedical Knowledge (MCBK)*. https://fci.org.uk/work-we-do/mcbk.html.

Health Education England (2021) *Knowledge for Healthcare: A Strategic Framework for NHS Knowledge and Library Services 2021–2026*. www.hee.nhs.uk/sites/default/files/documents/HEE%20Knowledge%20for%20Healthcare%202021-26%20FINAL.pdf.

Health Education England Knowledge and Library Services (2021a) *NHS Knowledge Mobilisation Framework*. https://library.hee.nhs.uk/knowledge-mobilisation/nhs-knowledge-mobilisation-framework-postcards.

Health Education England Knowledge and Library Services (2021b) *Knowledge Mobilisation Self-Assessment Tool*. https://library.hee.nhs.uk/knowledge-mobilisation/self-assessment-tool.

National Institute for Health Research (2013) New *Evidence on Management and Leadership*. www.journalslibrary.nihr.ac.uk/downloads/research-programmes/HSDR/New-Evidence-on-Management-and-Leadership.pdf.

NHS (2019) *The Topol Review: Preparing the Healthcare Workforce to Deliver the Digital Future – An Independent Report on Behalf of the Secretary of State for Health and Social Care*. https://topol.hee.nhs.uk/wp-content/uploads/HEE-Topol-Review-2019.pdf.

6

Internal and External Partnerships

Emily Hurt and Dawn Grundy

Introduction

Health Education England has acknowledged that there is a need to build and foster effective partnerships nationally and locally so that NHS library and knowledge services can ensure a consistent, equitable, funded core service to learners and staff and offer co-ordinated information to patients and the public (Health Education England, 2016). For public library services in England, Libraries Connected has a well established Universal Health Offer. This builds on the recognition of libraries as trusted spaces that deliver health information and recreational activities to help people better manage their health and wellbeing.

In effect, working with partners is an essential element of service delivery for information practitioners and healthcare decision makers. This chapter will explore the current context for cross-sector partnership working to help you identify potential internal and external partnerships within a health information setting, using case studies as examples. This will enable you to recognise the advantages that partnership working can bring to all involved. The chapter will also describe the key factors for effective partnership working, give some suggestions for implementing and embedding these and consider appropriate outcome measures to capture the impact of partnership working.

This chapter will help you think about partnership working in your current role and provide you with ideas about how to develop your skills and knowledge in this area. Throughout this chapter, we've included reflection points to help you think about how you would apply your learning in the real world. For more information on reflective practice and how it can be applied in librarianship see Chapter 11 and also Miller, Ford and Yang (2020).

Current context for cross-sector partnership working

Health Education England (2021) recognises the importance of cross-sector partnership working and the benefit this can have to individuals, organisations and society.

The two case studies discussed in this chapter illustrate this in practice. The first case study is based on an internal partnership within a trust setting and the second case study is a local partnership between differing organisations with a shared goal and interest in health and social care information.

Many educational or healthcare organisations will have a strategic vision discussing and documenting how they support communities' lifelong learning and encourage cross-sector working and collaboration to support and enhance the development of organisational goals and workforce knowledge and skills.

For example, the University of Bolton (2021) states: 'We will capitalise on our regional strength to build a national and international brand by enhancing the quality, reputation and perception of the organisation. This aim will be achieved through consolidation, focus, differentiation and the creation of the value through learning, teaching and knowledge exchange', which the Bolton Health Information Partnerships Memorandum of Understanding, ethos and practice supports and aligns to (see Case Study 6.2 below).

Keene and Downes (2020, 72) discuss library partnerships and how they can build a strong future for the library. The ever evolving world we live and work in influences partnership working, 'Inevitably therefore, library leaders are or will be increasingly required to work in partnership with others, even if not based in a joint library'.

In asking what partnership working is, Wildridge et al. (2004) acknowledge in their literature review that there is no one definition of partnership working and that it can be 'labelled' in several different ways, for example, as 'collaboration' or 'joint working'.

How to identify partners and case studies

One of the many attractions and incentives for working within the library and information sector is how collaborative and supportive organisations are. The desire to work in partnership, learn from others and share this good practice is intrinsic to our profession. Health libraries in particular have a strong 'do once and share' ethos and you'll find many collaborative working projects within the sector that have been written up as case studies or articles (for examples, see Carlyle, Thain and James, 2022; Irish et al., 2022; and Swanberg et al., 2022). Finding out about what others have done can help spark ideas for your own service.

Reflection point: Find some examples of partnership working case studies that have been written up in the literature. A good place to start looking might be the latest edition of *Information Professional* magazine or similar forums so you can learn from others within the sector. How were the partnerships established? What did they set out to do? Were they successful?

How to identify existing partnerships

If you're moving into a health library setting, there may well be established existing partnerships in place. Try to get an overview of who the service is already working with, both the internal and external partners. What was the original purpose of the partnership? Has the relationship developed and changed over time? Do any partnerships need refreshing – is there potential for a new project? Some partnerships may have lapsed, sometimes because a project has come to an end, but occasionally because of staff changes. The people who originally formed the partnership may have moved on to other roles and there is often a gap before a replacement is recruited. Are these lapsed partnerships worth rekindling?

You might want to use a table such as the one below to capture all the information you need. Once you've mapped out existing partnerships, it will help focus your next steps. It may be that you decide to concentrate on projects in hand and pause any new developments. Or the time might be right to do some horizon scanning and consider setting up a new partnership.

Table 6.1 *How to identify existing partnerships*

Partnership with (key people)	Date established	Initial aim	Key achievements	Future plans
Research and Innovation (Amanda James – R&I Nurse)	Nov 2019	To develop and deliver joint training programme to Occupational Therapy staff.	Delivered 20 workshops to date. Article in Trust newsletter. Increase in literature search requests from Occupational Therapists.	Repackage workshops and deliver to midwives.
Wards C3 and C4: Elderly Care (Carly Thwaite – Staff Nurse) Leytonshire Public Libraries (Andy Driscoll – Reader Engagement Manager)	Aug 2021	To provide Kindles with large print e-books preloaded for inpatients to use.	Four Kindles purchased with charitable funds. Four ward library accounts created so that books can be downloaded. Patient satisfaction increased.	Work with two new wards. Public library to recruit an e-book volunteer to visit wards and raise awareness/help inpatients use the service.

How to identify potential partnerships

Often, you won't need to go looking for new partnerships, they'll come to you – maybe through a chance conversation at a meeting or an email discussion. These naturally evolving partnerships can stem from a shared interest in developing a service, the identification of a problem that needs solving or a quality improvement project that could benefit from library involvement.

If a new potential partnership hasn't landed at your feet and you're actively looking to set something up to develop your service, there are a few things you can think about to help identify who you might involve:

- Gaps in your service – do you have a group of people you're not reaching?
- Trust-wide initiatives – is there something that your organisation is prioritising that you could tap into?
- National initiatives – campaigns such as Health Information Week or Libraries Week (2022) can provide you with an opportunity to work with another library or libraries (Linsey, 2020).
- Parallel departments – within an NHS setting there are other departments that sit outside of clinical areas and they often share the same potential customers as libraries (Human Resources, Organisational Development, Wellbeing Teams, Research, etc.).

If you can find something from the points above to base your partnership on, you stand a better chance of achieving real impact. Setting up a multi-party working group for the sake of ticking a 'collaborative working' box is likely to lead to directionless meetings and feelings of time better spent elsewhere (Libraries Connected, 2021a, 2).

Stakeholder analysis

Once your partnership is established and you have thought further about what you'd like to achieve, you may find it useful to carry out a stakeholder analysis. This can help you map out who has an interest in the work you are doing, how best to keep them updated and think about any specific risks you need to consider. Your stakeholders aren't just the people directly involved in your partnership – they could be groups that will be affected by the work your partnership is doing or individuals you are directly connected to, such as your line manager. A well executed analysis should enable you to manage your relationships and communicate with your stakeholders in a timely way.

Reflection point: Do some reading around stakeholder analysis models and find some worked examples online to familarise yourself with the exercise. A good starting point is the toolkit provided by NHS England and NHS Improvement (2022). There are others available on business websites – think how they would work with a library partnership.

Case studies
The following case studies are designed to illustrate how internal and external partnerships can be fostered and offer real-world advice and tips for establishing partnerships and the management and maintenance of them. We also reflect on challenges you may come across within partnership working and offer some tips on how to resolve those.

Case Study 6.1: Research Engagement Programme
The Research Engagement Programme was the result of an internal partnership between a clinical librarian and a research nurse at Lancashire Teaching Hospitals NHS Foundation Trust in 2016 (Hurt and McLoughlin, 2021). The two departments shared a similar position within the Trust as they were on the periphery of clinical activity and both physically located away from the main hospital building and had similar target audiences. The research nurse was part of the Clinical Academic Faculty within Research and Innovation (R&I), a small team responsible for increasing research capacity and capability amongst nurses, midwives and allied health professionals. The clinical librarian led a small team within Knowledge and Library Services (KLS) and was tasked with delivering information skills training as part of her role.

The two staff members met when the research nurse was asked to deliver a presentation about her work at a regional network meeting of clinical librarians. Realising they had a lot in common, they arranged a further meeting to talk about their current priorities and think about how they could work together. It soon became clear that delivering a joint training programme would bring benefits to both departments. R&I wanted to increase skills, knowledge and confidence with regards to research and KLS wanted to facilitate access to resources and help clinical staff find, evaluate and apply evidence in order to improve their practice.

Rather than offer a series of pre-specified workshops to all staff, a specific group was chosen (diagnostic radiographers) and all staff interested in taking part were given a choice of different workshops that they then voted for. The six most popular were developed and delivered. The team successfully applied for a research bursary from the CILIP Information Literacy Group and this in part paid for extra hours each week for both the research nurse and the clinical librarian. Both worked part time and the funding helped create time and space for developmental work to be carried out, rather than trying to shoehorn tasks into an already busy and pressured working week.

Following on from the initial delivery with diagnostic radiographers, the format of the programme was successfully repeated with therapeutic radiographers. The partnership stalled when the research nurse left the Trust to take up a post elsewhere, but the relationship between R&I and KLS was by that point well established and the two departments continued to involve each other in their work where possible. The appointment of a replacement member of staff meant that the partnership could be revitalised and the workshops delivered again, this time to advanced clinical practitioners and in a slightly different format as they were online rather than face-to-face.

One of the key objectives for the project was to create lesson plans and learning materials that other KLS and R&I departments could adapt and reuse. The intention was to inspire similar partnerships in other NHS Trusts and provide building blocks so that setting up future joint projects would require less work initially.

Case Study 6.2: Bolton Health Information Partnership

Bolton Health Information Partnership (BHIP) was formed in 2017, bringing together representatives from Bolton Library and Museum Services, Macmillan Cancer Information Services, Bolton NHS Foundation Trust Library Services and University of Bolton Library.

Informal partnerships were already in place historically between these organisations (Grundy, Elliott, and Stevens, 2019) but a new impetus to work together came with Health Information Week and the Knowledge for Healthcare initiative 'Developing and Building Local Networks and Partnerships', which sought to bring together local library services across a range of organisations to provide health information alongside Libraries Connected's Universal Library Offer 'Health and Wellbeing':

> Through the Health and Wellbeing Offer, libraries promote healthy living, provide self-management support and engagement opportunities for children and adults supported by welcoming spaces; effective signposting and information to reduce health, social and economic inequalities.
>
> (Libraries Connected, 2021b)

The formation of the Partnership offered an opportunity to share good practice across sectors and work together in the shared aim of helping people in Bolton with their health and wellbeing. The Partnership set up a Memorandum of Understanding (MoU), using Health Education England's guidance, that detailed the group's aims and objectives.

In addition to the main aim of the Partnership, all members of the group have shared aims and objectives, as well as clear roles and responsibilities for each organisation.

Shared aims and objectives
- To promote the importance of health literacy, including functional personalised information, which all people can make sense of and act on, to assist them to make informed choices, share in decisions about their care and treatment, take control and improve the quality of their life.
- To share and communicate good practice.

All parties also agree:

- to operate as strategic partners, looking for suitable opportunities to promote the aims stated in the MoU
- to work together on an increased evidence base to support these aims and objectives
- to work with partners to share guidance, good practice, expertise, experience and resources
- to facilitate/co-ordinate mutual training opportunities
- to work on joint projects and events, such as Health Information Week
- that any formal or detailed arrangements developed to implement joint actions through this agreement will be recorded and shared through the respective reporting arrangements to ensure that appropriate governance is established and good practice is cascaded.

These will include:

- development of any structural relationships
- building the evidence base
- nominating an alternative contact person if the named lead changes.

The roles and responsibilities listed in the MoU are guided by organisational, service and stakeholder needs; for example, a university would focus its remit on its community of staff and students, whereas a public library and museum service would look at the needs of a wider community.

Health Education England (2021) discusses the role that cross-sector partnerships can have in empowering health literate citizens:

> The community setting is the ideal place to develop the health literacy skills of the public. In our digital age, these skills must be underpinned by digital navigation. Information providers in the community include public libraries, college and education libraries, pharmacies, third sector organisations and prison libraries.
>
> (Health Education England, 2021)

Health Information Week

Since the Partnership's formation in 2017, Health Information Week is an activity that all the Bolton Health Information Partnership members can engage and contribute to. Health Information Week is a national, multi-sector campaign supporting high quality information for patients and the public. Between 2017 and 2022, Bolton Health Information Partnership's engagement with Health Information Week has taken place in a variety of forums, both face-to-face and online. Between 2017 and 2019, the majority of the collaborative work took place via 'pop-up' events and displays to support Health Information Week in different locations, highlighting the different organisations within the Partnership and how they can support the needs of the local community. In 2020, when the COVID pandemic struck, events moved online, including using social media for awareness campaigns on Twitter and an online guide to Health Information Week produced by the University (University of Bolton, 2020). Regardless of the pivot to online activities during the pandemic, the ethos of sharing good practice and resources within the Partnership remained very active.

Collection management

Within Bolton Health Information Partnership, Bolton Libraries and Museum Services have shared insights into the Reading Well collections and Books on Prescription. This has helped shape the development of wellbeing collections at Bolton College and the University of Bolton.

Lifelong learning

The sharing of relevant training or resources for the benefit of the Partnership is a standard item on the agenda of any meeting. This is a great opportunity to share developments within each organisation and learn from each other. Bolton Library and Museum Services have shared insight around running reading groups with Partnership members. The University of Bolton has shared its award-winning skills portal LEAP Online, which is predominately open access and can support the development of digital literacy, research skills and wellbeing.

Access agreements

There are access agreements in place for libraries within the Partnership and the group highlight and signpost to these and other members of the Partnership's services or resources. For those members of the Partnership who do not have a library service but are involved in healthcare information in community settings, such as Bolton Community Volunteer Service or

Healthwatch, membership of the Partnership gives them a vital insight into what libraries and knowledge services can offer.

Health Education England (2021) recognises the value of partnership working to enhance health literacy awareness (see Figure 6.1).

Strategic Outomes
- Staff, learners, patients and the public are better equipped to use evidence-based patient, health and wellbeing information for shared decision-making and self-care

Specific Outomes
- Information providers across the wider system have health literacy awareness and use evidence-based sources of patient, health and wellbeing information

Interventions
- With partners improve the health literacy awareness and digital literacy skills, including digital navigation, of the health and care workforce including learners
- Work with information providers to improve the health and digital literacy skills, including digital navigation, in community settings such as public libraries, prisons and schools
- Work with information providers to increase public access to evidence-based patient, health and wellbeing information

Figure 6.1 *Adapted from Health Education England,* Knowledge for Healthcare, *Health Literacy and Patient Information: Strategic Approach, 36*

Challenges within a partnership

Engagement within a partnership can be difficult to maintain. Creating an MoU or agreement within the parties regarding membership from each organisation will be crucial to a partnership's long-term success. It can help partners understand what they and others are contributing and the timescale involved and it can be used for accountability and sustainability purposes (Department for Education, 2022). If a member from an organisation leaves the partnership, who will replace them and carry on the work? Will there be a gap in expertise that could affect the aims and objectives of the partnership?

Health Education England acknowledges this and discusses strategic buy-in to support partnership working:

Partnership working is central to sharing best practice, optimising limited resources and reducing duplication. Excellent knowledge services require strategic buy-in, collaboration and commitment to maximise investment, nationally, locally and across health systems.

(Health Education England, 2021)

The benefits of working in collaboration or partnership to support individual knowledge and to support organisational objectives are clear. In the Bolton Health Information Partnership example (Case Study 6.2), the MoU between the members gave a strategic direction to the work of the Partnership to ensure continued collaboration and sharing of knowledge and good practice.

The advantages of partnership working

Leadership development

Working within, creating or leading a partnership can support new leadership development skills. Developing these skills with either internal or external partners can foster growth. The development of your leadership skills should give you an opportunity to reflect on:

- your own leadership style
- your project management skills
- the strategic context
- knowledge management.

Health Education England (2021) recognises the importance of workforce planning and development and its impact both on the profession and society (Figure 6.2 opposite).

> *Reflection point*: Think about how you have used your leadership skills in the past. What lessons have you learned and how could partnership working help develop your skills further? You could use the CILIP Professional Skills and Knowledge Base (PKSB) to identify any skills gaps you may have. The PKSB for the healthcare sector has been developed in partnership with Health Education England.

Community insight

Working within the healthcare sector offers opportunities to learn about the community and their needs and how we can support these as health information professionals. The definition of 'the community' can be

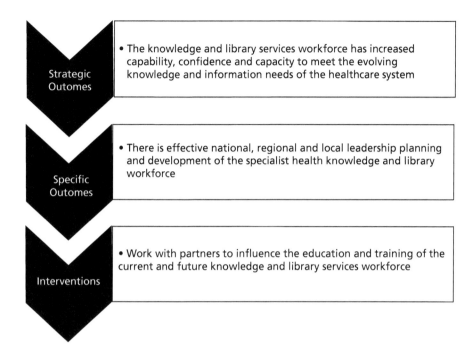

Figure 6.2 *Adapted from Health Education England,* Knowledge for Healthcare, *Health Literacy and Patient Information: Strategic Approach, 36*

interpreted in many ways: it may span different sectors or work across the organisation as seen in the two case studies above. We can act as advocates in terms of empowering knowledge across our communities. Health Education England (2021) acknowledges the importance of this role in ensuring we develop health literate citizens and equity of access to services across communities.

Effective partnership working requires an awareness of wider contexts; not just seeing things from the point of view of your organisation but considering the aims and objectives of others. Joining forces can lead to a better understanding of your community, both internal and external. It can break down barriers and reduce silo working where people, teams and organisations work towards the same objectives without realising, leading to duplication of effort.

Knowledge mobilisation

Partnership working naturally leads to the sharing of knowledge. Knowledge mobilisation is key to improving patient care and service delivery and information professionals are in an optimum position to facilitate the movement of knowledge. An effective partnership will involve sharing best practice, the creation and dissemination of new knowledge and the consolidation and summarising of existing knowledge.

The key factors for effective partnership working

Throughout this chapter, we discuss some of the factors for effective partnership working, using the case studies as practical examples and referencing national drivers to set the strategic context. The following are what we would determine as the key factors to success.

A Memorandum of Understanding or Terms of Reference for the partnership

This helps guide the remit of the group, demonstrates commitment and will also support changes in personnel within the group. It can also help develop learning for new members of the group or partnership as they join. Ideally, Memorandums of Understanding or Terms of Reference should be reviewed regularly to ensure the partnership is meeting its original purpose and/or aims and objectives.

Shared visions and goals

Discussing and analysing the partnership's shared visions and goals will help build mutual growth and understanding and strengthen working relationships.

Skills and knowledge

How will the partnership tap into the different skills and knowledge of the personnel or organisations within the group? Can one partner have increased impact in a particular area of the partnership for example? How will you develop as a 'team'?

Practical considerations

A 'home/platform'

Think about a formal place to share a brief biography and the activities of the partnership. Where is the most appropriate place for this? Potential spaces include a wiki, a blog, a page on an existing library website or on a regional library and knowledge services page as a partnership/community of practice section. Does any of the information need to be external or could it be hosted on an intranet? Would a social media account be beneficial to share the activities of the partnership? If so, who will manage and maintain it?

How will you meet and how often?
Meeting online can be advantageous for partnerships, particularly those in wider geographical locations, but consider the benefits of also meeting face-to-face if at all possible. Minutes of meetings should be kept and made available to all involved. This provides a record of decisions taken and actions allocated to group members. Even if your partnership is made up of two people, perhaps yourself and a colleague from another department, get into the habit of keeping notes whenever you meet. Trying to remember six months down the line why you decided on something can be tricky! Notes will also help you update your line manager on progress and actions taken.

Consider having meetings to complete a specific task, for example, where a workshop session plan is drafted or a project report is edited. Make the most of everyone in the partnership being in the same room for a couple of hours – those opportunities are rare and can prove very productive. If not everyone is able to attend, ensure that those absent have a chance to contribute or pass comment on key issues. Partnerships should involve everyone having an equal say.

Reflection point: From your own perspective, do you prefer meeting online or face-to-face? What do you feel are the advantages of either approach?

Outcome measures to capture the impact of partnership working

Ideally, you would think about impact measures sooner rather than later. It isn't always possible to capture the 'before' and 'after' with partnership working, but if you can collect some data around the status quo prior to work starting, this will help quantify what you've achieved further down the line. Sometimes this isn't feasible and so thinking about what you would like to measure as impact is the next best step. There may be multiple measures you could use, all of which could serve different purposes.

Imagine we are working with a staff nurse to provide Kindles to two elderly care wards in partnership with a reader engagement manager in public libraries. The main aim of the project is to increase patient satisfaction on the wards. This implies that patient satisfaction levels have already been measured, so the obvious action would be to measure them again after the project was up and running. But if we think about it further, there are other pieces of information we could collect that would demonstrate impact, both qualitative and quantitative:

- Number of patients who used the Kindles
- Number of e-books downloaded
- Number of patients who went on to use e-books after they were discharged from hospital
- Inpatient experience of patients who used the Kindles, collected through interview
- Project experience of the nurses and healthcare assistants who work on the ward, collected through interview.

We need to be prepared for negative as well as positive impact. If we asked the nurses and healthcare assistants about their experiences, they might say they found it time-consuming showing patients how to use the Kindles. Patient satisfaction might be greatly increased, but the ward found the project wasn't feasible due to time constraints. We can use this information to improve the project – for example, we might introduce trained volunteers to help patients rather than taking up the time of clinical staff.

Metrics

Other examples of measures to capture the impact of a partnership could include quantitative data, such as web page views. In the Bolton Health Information Partnership example above (Case Study 6.2), a library blog post that was published by University of Bolton Library detailing the Partnership's plans for Health Information Week in 2021 received a high number of web page hits and was also nominated for the LILAC FestivIL of Libraries award. A useful place to develop your knowledge and understanding of metrics is the Value and Impact Toolkit (Health Education England, 2022)

> *Reflection point*: How will you share the work of your partnership? If you've mapped out the stakeholders for your partnership, it may be that you need to communicate with them in different ways. Some may want a formal report on a regular basis, whereas communicating your work to a patient group would probably involve a newsletter article or a presentation to a group meeting.

Internal forums

How will you formally capture and share your impact? Will you include it in formal recording mechanisms for your organisation, such as an Annual Plan? Will you share the minutes of meetings with colleagues?

External forums
Will you write any outcomes or events up in a sector publication, such as *Information Professional*, or a newsletter, such as *Northern Lights*? Or will you present at a conference, such as a Health Libraries Group workshop or CILIP Conference?

Summary
Health Education England states:

> Collaboration is a guiding principle of our approach. Working with colleagues, with partner organisations and across the library, knowledge and information profession, we have made considerable progress – together inspired to harness our expertise and resources to common purpose.
>
> (Health Education England, 2021)

The case studies discussed in this chapter will help you understand internal and external partnerships and the benefits they can provide to individuals, services, organisations and the wider community. Partnerships can be complex to manage and keep on track, but with good planning, leadership and organisation, they offer a great opportunity to develop your knowledge and demonstrate your impact.

References
Carlyle, R., Thain, A. and James, S. (2022) Development and Spread of Health Literacy eLearning: A Partnership Across Scotland and England, *Health Information and Libraries Journal*, **39** (3), 299–303. https://doi.org/10.1111/hir.12450.

Department for Education (2022) *Guide to Writing a Memorandum of Understanding (MOU)*. www.gov.uk/government/publications/setting-up-school-partnerships/guide-to-writing-a-memorandum-of-understanding-mou.

Grundy, D., Elliott, P. and Stevens, A. (2019) Bolton Health Information Partnership, *Information Professional*, Oct–Nov, 24–6. http://ubir.bolton.ac.uk/2616.

Health Education England (2016) *NHS Library and Knowledge Services in England Policy*. www.hee.nhs.uk/sites/default/files/documents/NHS Library and Knowledge Services in England Policy.pdf.

Health Education England (2021) *Knowledge for Healthcare: Mobilising Evidence; Sharing Knowledge; Improving Outcomes. A Strategic Framework for NHS Knowledge and Library Services 2021–2026*. www.hee.nhs.uk/our-work/knowledge-for-healthcare.

Health Education England (2022) *Metrics*. https://library.hee.nhs.uk/quality-and-impact/value-and-impact/value-and-impact-toolkit/metrics.

Health Information Week (2023) *Health Information Week*. https://healthinfoweek.wixsite.com/healthinfoweek.

Hurt, E. and McLoughlin, A. (2021) Facilitating Research Amongst Radiographers Through Information Literacy Workshops, *Journal of the Medical Library Association*, **109** (1), 112–19. https://doi.org/10.5195/jmla.2021.842.

Irish, E., Burke, K., Geyer, E. and Allard, I. (2022) Patient Empowerment: A Partnership for Community Engagement in Three Phases, *Journal of Consumer Health on the Internet*, **26** (1), 109–18. https://doi.org/10.1080/15398285.2022.2030143.

Keene, J. and Downes, J. (2020) Do Library Partnerships Work and How Can They Help Build a Strong Future for the Library? In Weaver, M. and Appleton, L. (eds), *Bold Minds: Library Leadership in a Time of Disruption*, Facet Publishing.

Libraries Connected (2021a) *Expert Bank: Partnership Toolkit*. www.librariesconnected.org.uk/resource/expert-bank-partnership-toolkit.

Libraries Connected (2021b) *Universal Library Offers, Health and Wellbeing*. www.librariesconnected.org.uk/universal-offers/health-wellbeing.

Libraries Week (2022) *Libraries Week*. http://librariesweek.org.uk.

Linsey, S. (2020) *Partnership Working with Public Libraries – Health Information Covid-19 and Beyond*. https://library.hee.nhs.uk/about/blogs/partnership-working-with-public-libraries--health-.

Miller, J., Ford, S. and Yang, A. (2020) Elevation Through Reflection: Closing the Circle to Improve Librarianship, *Journal of the Medical Library Association*, **108** (1), 353–63. https://jmla.pitt.edu/ojs/jmla/article/view/938.

NHS England and NHS Improvement (2022) *Quality, Service Improvement and Redesign Tools: Stakeholder Analysis*. www.england.nhs.uk/wp-content/uploads/2022/02/qsir-stakeholder-analysis.pdf.

Swanberg, S. M., Bulgarelli, N., Jayakumar, M., Look, E., Wedemeyer, R., Yuen, E. W. and Lucia, V. C. (2022) A Health Education Outreach Partnership Between an Academic Medical Library and Public Library: Lessons Learned Before and During a Pandemic, *Journal of the Medical Library Association*, **110** (2), 212–21. https://doi.org/10.5195/jmla.2022.1413.

University of Bolton (2020) *Health Information Week 2020*. https://libguides.bolton.ac.uk/lifelounge/healthinfoweek.

University of Bolton (2021) *University Strategy.* www.bolton.ac.uk/welcome-to-hr/university-strategy.

Wildridge, V., Childs, S., Cawthra, L. and Madge, B. (2004) How to Create Successful Partnerships – A Review of the Literature, *Health Information and Libraries Journal,* **21** (s1), 3–19.

7

Health Literacy, Patient Information and Combating Misinformation

Joanne Naughton and Geoff Walton

Introduction

In this chapter, we explore definitions of health literacy in relation to individuals and wider society. We will examine which groups in society are more likely to be affected by low health literacy and describe how having low health literacy impacts on a person's health and wellbeing and the services that support them. We'll also set out tools and techniques that can help people with low health literacy and promote health literacy in practice. Finally, we outline the context for work by health library and knowledge specialists in promoting health literacy.

What is health literacy?

Health literacy can be defined in relation to an individual and to wider society.

Individuals

For an individual, health literacy describes the extent to which a person can find, understand, use and apply health information as well as interact with healthcare services to make health-related choices for themselves and others. Health information behaviour and health literacy are complex phenomena that have received much attention in information behaviour research, such as how people engage with or avoid health information (Saironen and Savolainen, 2010). Critical health literacy (Sykes et al., 2013) is one notion that has been employed to empower individuals to make informed decisions. However, information behaviour research demonstrates that whilst some individuals will readily seek health information, some will actually actively avoid it in order to reduce the risk of experiencing negative emotions such as fear, anxiety and depression (Saironen and Savolainen, 2010; Case and Given, 2016). Although the vast majority of people will seek health information to reduce anxiety, for some, engaging with health information can increase their anxiety (Pifalo et al., 1997).

Society

For a society or healthcare system, health literacy relates to the provision of information and services in a way that is accessible to all and empowers people to make informed healthcare decisions. However, the COVID pandemic and the scare regarding the link between the Measles Mumps and Rubella (MMR) vaccine and autism (Lewandowsky et al., 2012) have put into stark relief how health misinformation can spread, often quicker than good quality information (Spring, 2020). The term 'infodemic' aptly describes the former phenomenon (Zaracostas, 2020). What we can conclude from this is that, as health information professionals, it isn't simply a question of providing good quality health information, there is also a need to actively combat misinformation and deliberate disinformation which is so easily available via the internet.

The dual aspect of health literacy (individual and societal) is reflected in the World Health Organization definition:

> Health literacy refers to the personal characteristics and social resources needed for individuals and communities to access, understand, appraise and use information and services to make decisions about health.
>
> (Dodson, Good and Osborne, 2015)

To overcome the individual and societal health literacy problems and to improve health literacy, it is clear that action is required to help people to develop their personal health literacy skills and, at the same time, ensure that the NHS and the wider health and care system provides good quality health information that can be accessed and understood by everyone who needs it. The availability of good quality information and positive health conversations will in turn help people to increase their confidence and knowledge and is likely to lead to better engagement in their own healthcare. As one GP explains: 'Time spent supporting my patients to develop language and confidence in health pays dividends in supporting their health and their self-management of illness' (GP working in a deprived city practice in the north east of England, personal communication, 3 March 2022). An important part of healthcare engagement is shared decision-making, where a healthcare professional and an individual agree an approach to treatment or managing a health condition. In some national policies, such as shared decision-making in England and Wales, health literacy skills are specifically referenced (NICE, 2021).

How many people are affected by low health literacy?

In England, 43% of working age adults are unable to understand and make use of everyday health information, rising to 61% when numeracy skills are needed for understanding (Rowlands et al., 2015). This indicates that health information is too complex for most of us to understand.

Who is more likely to be affected by low health literacy?

Certain population groups are more at risk of limited health literacy (Public Health England, 2015). These groups include:

- people from disadvantaged socioeconomic groups
- migrants and people from ethnic minorities
- older people
- people with long-term conditions
- disabled people.

Research in the US (Paasche-Orlow et al., 2005; Rudd, 2007) and the EU (Sorensen et al., 2015) found similar results, with educational level as an additional factor. Characterised by some as 'information poverty' (Case and Given, 2016), this phenomenon appears to be a reflection of social inequality and is manifest in terms of a low level of processing skills, such as reading, social isolation and a fatalistic outlook. It is linked to information avoidance where those with low levels of processing skills feel a sense of information overload that causes them anxiety and hence they avoid the information altogether. To begin to address this issue, Health Education England commissioned the development of a health literacy data site that uses survey data on literacy and numeracy as a measure of health literacy levels at the local authority level in England (University of Southampton, 2020). This geodata site can help to target priority areas for health literacy interventions. It is also a useful training tool as it helps health and care professionals to relate to health literacy needs in their local area.

Why does low health literacy matter?

There is evidence to show that limited health literacy is linked to poorer health outcomes (Baker et al., 2002; Cho et al., 2008) and higher mortality rates (Wolf et al., 2010). Those with lower health literacy levels are less likely to take up screening appointments or to have a healthy lifestyle, for example, healthy eating (von Wagner et al., 2007; Chen et al., 2013; Chesser et al., 2016). Information literacy research by Walton et al. (2022) also found that those less able to make good judgements about information ('information discernment') were at risk of experiencing a negative stress reaction to misinformation. The implication of this is that, when encountering health misinformation, those with low levels of health literacy may be vulnerable to experiencing an additional negative effect on their physiological wellbeing. In other words, health literacy is a key determinant of health.

Improving health literacy has the potential to empower people to build their confidence and skills in order to take more control of their own health and wellbeing and reduce risks to health. Developing health literacy skills can form part of a wider strategy to reduce health inequalities.

Digital health literacy

Health information and interactions are increasingly digital. However, 2.6 million people living in the UK are still offline and one-third of benefit claimants have very low digital engagement (Lloyds Bank, 2021). People with low health digital literacy skills can be particularly vulnerable to misleading health information. We also know that meeting the health information needs of people who are marginalised or disadvantaged can help to reduce health inequality (Gann, 2020).

Health literacy in a pandemic

> Covid has been a real crash course in a health literacy experience on a planetary scale.
>
> (Guinn Delaney, cited in Economist Intelligence Unit, 2021, 55)

Higher levels of health literacy can help to reduce pressure on healthcare systems and lead to behaviours that promote public health. For this reason, improving health literacy is an important means of addressing health challenges such as pandemics and the related 'infodemic' identified by Zaracostas (2020).

Levels of health literacy

Health literacy is difficult to measure in terms of skills/achievements. Don Nutbeam (2000) adapted existing literacy models to describe health literacy in terms of what our skills allow us to do:

- Level 1: **Functional health literacy**: the skills to be able to function with day-to-day health information, for example, read leaflets, labels and to understand basic verbal health communication.
- Level 2: **Interactive health literacy**: more advanced cognitive, literacy and social skills that allow us to interact with a range of health information as an active participant, applying information to new situations.
- Level 3: **Critical health literacy**: more advanced literacy, cognitive and social skills allowing us to critically review a range of types of

information, to interact with and challenge the healthcare system and exert control over health outcomes.

Reflection point: How is your health literacy? Consider how receptive you are to health information. How do you rate your confidence and skill in understanding and managing health information?

- Right now, in a work or study context.
- When supporting a loved one.
- When diagnosed with a life-changing condition.

What are the factors that affect your health literacy?

Why does health literacy change?
Poor health literacy is not just about having low skills, although this is one of the most basic barriers to good health literacy.

Most people will have health literacy needs at some time during their life, regardless of their skills level (McKenna, Sixsmith and Barry, 2017):

- when managing multiple/new health conditions
- because healthcare/illness can be a frightening thing for many people
- the language of health can be unfamiliar to people
- because there is often stress and anxiety associated with health, for example, existing illness, new diagnosis.

What is the impact of low health literacy?
For the NHS
Low health literacy is costly for the NHS and for any healthcare system. One study estimated that limited reading and numeracy-related health literacy accounted for an additional 3 to 5% of total healthcare cost annually (National Academy on an Ageing Society, 1999).

Improving access to health information and enabling patients to take an active role in their own health and wellbeing brings financial benefits to the healthcare system in terms of reducing wasted medications, demand for GP appointments, A&E attendances, emergency admissions, re-admissions and the amount of time spent in hospital, as well as reducing compensation and legal costs (Patient Information Forum, 2013, 13).

For patients, the public and healthcare staff
Health literacy stories
Here are some real examples of misunderstandings that result from low health literacy and/or poor health communication. Consider the impact of these misunderstandings for the people concerned in terms of their wellbeing and ability to manage their own health:

- A woman who sprayed her inhaler on her dog as she had learned that she was allergic to her dog.
- A man who thought the progression of his tumour was a good thing.
- A woman turning back from an oncology centre as she had been told to go to the cancer centre.

These stories show us that health literacy is a real issue with damaging and sometimes dangerous consequences for people who use the services and for the staff who support them.

What is the role of NHS knowledge and library specialists?
Knowledge for Healthcare is the Health Education England Strategic Framework that shapes the work of knowledge and library specialists in England. Our strategic ambition is that:

> NHS bodies, their staff, learners, patients and the public use the right knowledge and evidence, at the right time, in the right place, enabling high quality decision-making, learning, research and innovation to achieve excellent healthcare and health improvement.
>
> (Health Education England, 2021, 6)

NHS knowledge specialists are based in a range of different settings (mental health services, community and hospitals) and work in varied and imaginative ways to improve the experience of patients, carers and service users. Some services have created bespoke resources for patients, for example, reminiscence boxes for dementia patients, and these resources can be used on wards and sometimes in the library, depending on the organisation. Some librarians work directly with patients, helping them to find health information or even running reading groups with them. Other services have trained local public librarians in the skills they need to manage health enquiries in the community.

Health librarians are recognised as experts in facilitating access to high quality research evidence and knowledge for healthcare staff. They are skilled in finding, appraising, organising and structuring health information. NHS knowledge specialists provide evidence summaries and syntheses to inform patient care, service planning and policymaking within the health service. Increasingly, knowledge specialists provide summaries of evidence to inform patient information. Some services also manage the process of updating patient leaflets (print and digital), using their information management skills to ensure that patient information is evidence-based, systematically updated and delivered in a consistent, accessible format for everyone who needs it.

As information literacy experts who work closely with other healthcare professionals, NHS knowledge specialists are natural champions of the health literacy 'movement'. Since 2018, Health Education England (working initially with the Community Health and Learning Foundation) has been delivering a programme of health literacy awareness training to NHS knowledge and library specialists and some library specialists from other relevant fields, for example, public libraries and higher education. The training covers much of the content discussed in this chapter, including the impact of low health literacy for the individual and the healthcare system and tools and techniques to improve health literacy and simplify information.

Based on evaluation data from early in the delivery of the health literacy programme, Health Education England worked with partners to develop and promote a range of learning materials to suit different learning styles, training scenarios and audiences. As a short introduction to health literacy, the eLearning for Healthcare Health Literacy Programme (NHS Education for Scotland and Health Education England, 2020) gives a good overview of the impacts and provides signposts to tools to help. A 15-minute, bitesize face-to-face session was developed for use in inductions or as a short taster to stimulate interest. For trainers with more time, a one-hour session was made available and was accredited by the Royal Society for Public Health. When training was delivered face-to-face, the full health literacy awareness and train the trainer programme involved one-day sessions and were delivered at the regional level. Since the COVID pandemic, the training has been delivered as a half-day online. The *NHS England Health Literacy Toolkit* (2023) provides a useful toolkit to support training delivery.

At the time of writing, 264 knowledge specialists have gone through the awareness training, out of which 61 are now active trained trainers with the skills to cascade this training to others. These trainers have cascaded to over 300 healthcare professionals within the NHS. There is strong engagement in the wider healthcare system and Health Education England is responding by increasing capacity to deliver training to meet growing demand. There is a thriving, national health literacy community of practice where knowledge specialists with varying degrees of expertise and knowledge share resources and know-how. The focus of this group is on developing skills and confidence in training delivery among knowledge specialists.

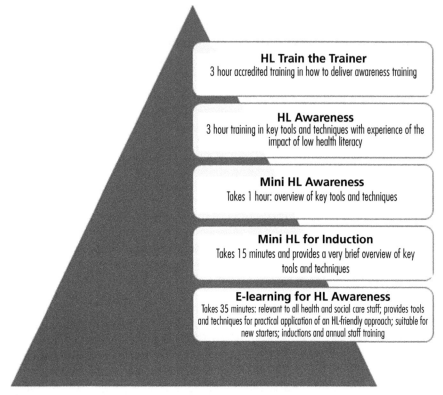

Figure 7.1 *Model for scale and spread of health literacy training*, adapted from Ruth Carlyle and Sally James, *Health Education England*, 2019

Health literacy in practice

Here are examples of how NHS knowledge and library services are making an impact on health literacy awareness and action in their own organisations and communities.

Case Study 7.1: Collaborative working with public library

Team/project lead: North East London NHS Foundation Trust / Catherine Jenkins
Trust: North East London NHS Foundation Trust
Target group: The public
Library specialists from the Mental Health Trust worked closely with public library colleagues to deliver drop-in health information sessions for the public as part of the Universal Health Offer.

'Allows people to access and be signposted to up-to-date information by specialists – we don't have that capability', Development Librarian, Redbridge Public Libraries.

NHS knowledge and library specialists also worked with a local Children and Adolescent Mental Health Services (CAMHS) to provide access to the Reading Agency Shelf Help Collection (specifically designed to support younger people with mental health issues). They helped to design display materials and the collection has been promoted and used effectively by the team. One team member, who works with young offenders, described how one client with low literacy skills responded when she read aloud to him from one of the books:

'So every session we had, we'd have a little bit of time talking about where he was with his mental health, and then we'd sit and go "OK, Jackanory Time", and I'd spend half an hour reading him this book.'

While the book was being read to him, her client turned up for every single session, was much more engaged and achieved better outcomes in treatment: 'And he would sit there and he would suddenly say, "Oh yeah, I get that!" "Yes that's me!" "I really understand it!"'

Key themes: relationship building, health information, mental health

Case Study 7.2: Health literacy and health misinformation training

Team/project lead: Greater Manchester Mental Health NHS Foundation Trust / Lorna Dawson
Trust: Greater Manchester Mental Health NHS Foundation Trust
Target group: Health and social care staff

At Greater Manchester Mental Health NHS Foundation Trust, the Library and Knowledge Service team delivers the Better Information Programme, which offers Health Literacy Awareness and Introduction to Misinformation training.

The Health Literacy course raises awareness of poor health literacy levels in Manchester and signposts to techniques to improve written and verbal health literacy communication. The Misinformation course teaches attendees how to check the quality of online health information and spot the signs of misinformation.

The training is delivered to staff in health, social care, community and voluntary organisations across Manchester. It uses a cascade model where attendees are encouraged to share the training with colleagues as well as their users.

The training was particularly popular during the COVID pandemic when misinformation was rife and when it was also evident that health literacy barriers stopped certain populations receiving important COVID updates, for example, people with English as a second language.

A Volunteer Co-ordinator at the COVID-19 Chat Community Champions programme shared how the training has helped prevent the spread of misinformation and fraud:

'After the training I came across a supposed government link that was being circulated on WhatsApp and social media to help people who had contracted COVID and needed assistance accessing financial support from the NHS Test and Trace team. Ordinarily after seeing a post with the government logo, I would immediately share with my network and people in the community without checking its authenticity, but on this occasion, I decided to subject the post to a test from the training called the SHARE checklist, and this test helped me avoid sharing a link which was a scam to defraud unsuspecting people in the community.'

Key themes: health information and misinformation, mental health

Case Study 7.3: Health literacy awareness training

Team/project lead: Northern Devon Healthcare NHS Trust / Lynsey Southern
Trust: Northern Devon Healthcare NHS Trust
Target group: Healthcare professionals

Health literacy offers an opportunity to extend the skill set of the healthcare librarian. In my role as an NHS Knowledge and Library Service (KLS) Manager, it is also the chance to develop my communication and teaching skills.

I've delivered sessions to junior doctors, preceptors, social prescribers, paramedics, GPs and student nurses. The reach of our health literacy offer is now moving into the community, where I support the development of a five-year community health inequalities strategic plan bringing our KLS health literacy expertise to the table.

Health literacy is often an unknown term when people attend their first session but its impact is far reaching on individuals and teams. The sharing of local health literacy levels is a shock but the practical skills training we deliver enables staff to catalyse the information and make an immediate change to their everyday practice.

Quotes from healthcare professionals who have attended health literacy training:

'The session helped me learn the importance of teach back and to use it effectively. It's taught me that I need to do things differently and to check my comprehension when discussing missed pills rules with patients.' – Preceptor
'I have gained knowledge and will be clearer with medications, specify medication times, doses, etc. To make sure that patients have clear information.' – Nurse
'The team here on ICU [Intensive Care Unit] are always very conscious of how distressing it can be to have a loved one admitted to the critical care

environment, and how intimidating and overwhelming it can be for visitors to see all of the equipment and attachments. We had been looking for a way to help alleviate some of the stresses for visitors to the environment by having a display with pictorial references and simple text to make the information accessible to all. After listening to our excellent librarian, Lynsey Southern, talk about health literacy and its importance and seeing other healthcare trusts tweeting about similar displays, I contacted a company who specialise in making healthcare infographic panels. We are delighted with the results.' – ICU team

Key themes: relationship building, seizing an opportunity, awareness raising, highlighting services and skills

Case Study 7.4: Health literacy champions

Team/project lead: Dorset County Hospital NHS Foundation Trust / Morag Evans
Trust: Dorset County Hospital NHS Foundation Trust
Target group: Healthcare staff
Health Literacy Awareness training has led to the setting up of health literacy champions in a trust in Dorset.

After attending health literacy awareness training, and with the help of a 'Plan, Do, Study, Act' approach, the librarian recruited several members of staff as health literacy champions who are passionate about raising awareness of and signposting good quality health information to both colleagues and patients. Champions meet every two months, with the librarian reporting monthly to the Trust's Health Inequalities Group. Training in health literacy is also delivered to doctors in their inductions and at preceptorship study days, as well as ad-hoc workshops for other members of staff. A bulletin on health literacy has also been produced. Evaluations are captured using Slido and used to inform future training. Health literacy awareness training has also encouraged library staff to demystify and simplify some of the terms used in library 'jargon', which has informed marketing strategies, displays and other promotional material produced. Further afield, the librarian has worked with the county's public library managers in delivering health literacy awareness, leading to further events and liaison with public library colleagues.

Key themes: relationship building, seizing an opportunity, health literacy training

Health literacy in the prison environment

Health Education England has been working in partnership with a group of prison librarians to address health literacy issues among the prison population. Prison librarians report that the single most important obstacle to accessing current, high quality health information for prisoners is digital access. Most prisoners have no access to online content (for security reasons). The disparity between wider society and prison, in terms of access to health information, is growing as health information and health consultations are increasingly made available digitally.

We know that those with lower literacy and numeracy skills suffer worse health outcomes. It is estimated that 50% of people in prisons have a reading age of 11 or below (Shannon Trust, 2022). Many have had negative educational experiences, low self-confidence and may lack motivation. Providing a safe environment with resources that are accessible and engaging is a constant challenge for prison librarians.

As part of the partnership, Health Education England delivered health literacy awareness and train the trainer sessions to prison librarians, who are now spotting opportunities to roll out health literacy training as part of their offer into prisons.

Health Education England facilitated links between prison librarians and local NHS knowledge and library services. These links have helped in terms of access to high quality health information and in providing opportunities for prison librarians to build confidence in their health literacy skills. The partnership with prison librarians is ongoing and a range of opportunities to improve health literacy are emerging including:

- building links with health professionals and education teams in the prison service
- making resources available via Prisons online platform, Virtual Campus and signposting staff
- developing a programme to promote the prison librarian's role in health literacy and patient information, using existing communication channels to engage prisoners/residents in their own health and wellbeing, for example, tailored health features in a prison magazine
- roll out of health literacy training to CILIP Prison Libraries Group
- opportunities to shadow NHS librarians
- developing impact case studies to showcase the contribution prison libraries make to health and wellbeing.

Partnerships in health literacy

As already described in this chapter, health literacy is multi-factoral and low health literacy can affect us all, at different times in our lives. Partnership approaches (see Chapter 6) are needed to address the range of societal, system and personal factors that can influence health literacy.

The National Health and Digital Literacy Partnership is a cross-sectoral initiative led by Health Education England and facilitated by CILIP. The aim of the Partnership is that citizens have the health literacy skills, the underpinning digital skills and resources to make shared decisions and manage their health and wellbeing.

Member organisations have signed a Compact that expresses a shared commitment to working together to establish a sustainable, common information environment through which skilled information providers, for example, library staff, pharmacists and third sector staff, support and empower digitally and health literate citizens.

There are three main strands to the work of the partnership:

- **Workstream 1** focuses on skills development for information providers and the public to develop their digital and digital health navigation skills and the development of tools and resources.
- **Workstream 2** cascades training and promotes access to high quality health information resources and tools, such as the Health Literacy Geodata Site (University of Southampton, 2020) and, in the longer term, a sustainable platform to host resources.
- **Workstream 3** involves building community partnerships and testing approaches through pilots to see what works well. Health Education England have funded a range of small community projects. These pilots have included: building community digital health hubs; funding health literacy training; health and digital literacy champion schemes; resource kits for outreach health; and digital literacy work with 16 to 25-year-olds. The partnership builds on existing infrastructure. The aim is to ensure sustainability by making health literacy part of digital skills, information skills and information service access in local communities.

Improving health literacy: some tools and techniques

Tools to help when speaking to patients, service users and carers

Teach back is an evidence-based technique recommended by NICE (2021) to ensure that patients and carers understand the information that has been given to them by asking them to explain what has been discussed in their own words. The healthcare professional takes responsibility for communicating the message clearly so that the burden is not on the patient. So, for example, a healthcare professional might say 'Just so I can be sure that I have explained everything clearly, could you please tell me how you will take this medication.'

Chunk and check means ensuring that you break information down into small, manageable chunks so that people can take in the information. Use this technique with teach back so you can check for understanding after giving a chunk of information (rather than waiting until the end) is most effective.

Keeping health information simple

Much of the information we receive about our health and wellbeing is in print and digital format. Given that the majority of the population struggle with everyday health information (Rowlands et al., 2015) and that 14.9% of adults in England read and write at or below the level we would expect of a 9 to 11-year-old (Department for Business, Innovation and Skills, 2012), it is important that all healthcare information is provided in simple, accessible language. There is a whole range of factors that affect how we can access and use written health information, including literacy, language skills and a range of disabilities (visible and hidden). The Accessible Information Standard (NHS England, 2016) is designed to set out a common approach to meeting the information needs of people with a disability, impairment or sensory loss. All organisations that provide NHS care and/or publicly funded adult social care are legally required to follow the Standard, which stipulates that health information must be provided in an accessible format, such as British Sign Language, where this is requested.

Free tools to simplify written language

There are a range of free tools to help to simplify language and assess the reading age of any written material. These include:

- Hemingway Editor
- SMOG Readability Formula
- Plain English Campaign.

Health information tools

- NHS Digital Content Style Guide: a guide for staff to produce accessible, inclusive health information.
- Ask 3 Questions Tool: designed to help patients and carers to make the most of their health appointments. Easy Read versions of these tools have been co-created by Health Education England in collaboration with IC Works and people with learning disabilities.

Finding good quality health information

The NHS website provides an A to Z Guide to treatments, symptoms and health and wellbeing information that covers most common conditions. Royal Colleges and third sector organisations also provide valuable specialist health information for a range of less common conditions on their websites, for example, Macmillan Cancer Support, Royal College of Obstetricians and Gynaecologists.

During the pandemic, the need to ensure access for all to reliable health information became even more important. NHS knowledge and library specialists responded by signposting high quality digital content from their websites. Health Education England created a Health and Coronavirus Information website.

There is a huge range of sources of health information available and the ability to differentiate between good and poor quality, or even dangerous content, is a key health and digital literacy skill. There are several tools that can help to judge the reliability of health information online:

- CRAAP Test: designed to assess the quality of any online information.
- DISCERN: quality criteria for consumer health information.
- SHARE Checklist: to help citizens decide what information it is safe to share online.

Exercises
How health literate is the NHS?
Read the following list of medical terms and abbreviations used commonly in NHS communications and signage. Take one minute to write down the meaning of the terms or any synonyms without the use of any tools to help:

Radiology
Acute
Gynaecological Oncology
Chronic
Hypertension
CT Scan
Colposcopy
Obstetrics
MRI Scan
Prosthetics
Phlebotomy

How far did you get?

Reflection and discussion
- How easy is it for the public to understand healthcare information and signage?

- What kind of issues might this cause for patients and the public?
- How could the healthcare system make it easier for people to understand health information and signage?

Using teach back and chunk and check to simplify spoken communication
Example: Preparing for surgery: eating and drinking
Nurse: So, Mr Smith, you will be having your surgery on Tuesday next week. It is very important that you stop eating and drinking in plenty of time before your surgery to give your stomach time to empty. This will help to avoid problems during surgery.

On Monday, you can eat and drink normally. Follow your normal routines up to 1 o'clock on Tuesday morning, so that is Monday night into Tuesday morning. You must eat nothing after 1 o'clock on Tuesday morning. So, just to make sure I have made this clear, can you tell me what time you will eat your last food before your surgery?

[Patient response....]

That's great. So for drinking, you must stop drinking tea, coffee, alcohol and any other drinks except water from 1 o'clock in the morning, so that is Monday night into Tuesday morning. You can still drink water but only until 6 o'clock on Tuesday morning. From 6 o'clock in the morning you must not drink anything.

Again, just so I can be sure I have explained these instructions clearly, can you tell me when you will have your last drink before surgery?

[Patient response....]

Note: this scenario does not represent clinical advice. It has been created for learning purposes only.

Group activity
Working in groups of three or four, decide who will be the patient, the clinician and the observer(s) for the clinical scenario.

1 The clinician reads the scenario and prepares an approach to sharing this information with a patient. The patient should not read the scenario.
2 Consider potential areas for confusion and how you would address these using spoken and written communication. Use teach back and chunk

and check methods to get your key messages across, keeping the burden of communication on you.
3   The patient can ask questions and tries to process the information, relying on the explanation of the health professional.
4   The observer notices what works well and what could work better and feeds back at the end of the practice.

Remember, keep your information and instructions clear and concise. This activity should take around 20 minutes to complete (including feedback).

Get some practice
Clinical scenario
You are prescribing metronizadole (an antibiotic) to a patient to treat a leg ulcer. How would you explain this information to a patient in plain language, using teach back and chunk and check to ensure understanding?
Here is the information you need to explain to the patient:

Dosage: 400 mg (2 x 200 mg tablets) every 8 hours.
Warning: Patient must avoid alcohol while taking the antibiotic and for 48 hours after they have finished the course – if alcohol is consumed, the patient may well experience a disulfiram-like reaction (nausea, vomiting, flushing, dizziness, throbbing headache, chest and abdominal discomfort, and tachycardia (fast heartbeat)).
Instructions:
Take with or just after food or a meal.
Swallow this medicine whole. Do not chew or crush.
Take with a full glass of water.
Space the doses evenly throughout the day.
Keep taking this medicine until the course is finished, unless you are told to stop.

Note: this scenario does not represent clinical advice. It has been created for learning purposes only.
(Information taken from the British National Formulary (2022) and Patient UK (2022).)

Consider:

• What were the main points noted by the observer(s)?
• What did you learn from this exercise?

- Can you see ways of applying teach back and chunk and check in different work or learning settings?

Summary and key learning points
- Health literacy is complex and is influenced by a range of factors (societal and personal).
- Low health literacy is a widespread problem and is related to health inequality.
- Even those with high levels of health literacy may struggle to find and use health information effectively during times of stress or illness.
- Low health literacy can have serious consequences for individuals and the healthcare system.
- There is a range of high quality tools to help to simplify information (both written and verbal).
- NHS knowledge and library specialists play a key role as health literacy advocates and in facilitating access to high quality health information for patients and the public.
- Partnership working with other information providers and specialists is essential for successful health literacy interventions.

Acknowledgements

Ruth Carlyle, Head of Knowledge and Library Services: Midlands, East and North of England, Health Education England.

Lorna Dawson, Public Health and Engagement Librarian, Greater Manchester Mental Health NHS Foundation Trust.

Morag Evans, Librarian, Dorset County Hospital NHS Foundation Trust.

Catherine Jenkins, Health Literacy Project Manager, North East London NHS Foundation Trust.

Lynsey Southern, Knowledge and Library Services Manager, Northern Devon Healthcare NHS Trust

References

Baker, D. W., Gazmararian, J. A., Williams, M. V., Scott, T., Parker, R. M., Green, D., Ren, J. and Peel, J. (2002) Functional Health Literacy and the Risk of Hospital Admission Among Medicare Managed Care Enrollees, *American Journal of Public Health*, **92** (8), 1278–83.

British National Formulary (2022) *Metronidazole*. https://bnf.nice.org.uk/drug/metronidazole.html#indicationsAndDoses.

Case, D. O. and Given, L. M. (2016) *Looking for Information: A Survey of Research on Information Seeking, Needs and Behavior* (4th edn), Emerald.

Chen, J. Z., Hsu, H. C., Tung, H. J. and Pan, L. Y. (2013) Effects of Health Literacy to Self-Efficacy and Preventive Care Utilization Among Older Adults, *Geriatrics and Gerontology International*, **13** (1), 70–6.

Chesser, A. K., Keene Woods, N., Smothers, K. and Rogers, N. (2016) Health Literacy and Older Adults: A Systematic Review, *Gerontology and Geriatric Medicine*, 2, (1–13).
https://journals.sagepub.com/doi/pdf/10.1177/2333721416630492.

Cho, Y. I., Lee, S. Y., Arozullah, A. M. and Crittenden, K. S. (2008) Effects of Health Literacy on Health Status and Health Service Utilisation Amongst the Elderly, *Social Science and Medicine*, **66** (8), 1809–16.

Department for Business, Innovation and Skills (2012) *The 2011 Skills for Life Survey: A Survey of Literacy, Numeracy and ICT Levels in England.*
www.gov.uk/government/publications/2011-skills-for-life-survey.

Dodson, S., Good, S. and Osborne, R. H. (2015) *Health Literacy Toolkit for Low and Middle-Income Countries: A Series of Information Sheets to Empower Communities and Strengthen Health Systems*, Information Sheet 1, World Health Organization.
https://apps.who.int/iris/handle/10665/205244.

Economist Intelligence Review Unit (2021) *Health Literacy Around the World: Policy Approaches to Wellbeing Through Knowledge and Empowerment.* https://eiuperspectives.economist.com/healthcare/health-literacy-around-world-policy-approaches-wellbeing-through-knowledge-and-empowerment.

Gann, B. (2020) Combating Digital Health Inequality in the Time of Coronavirus, *Journal of Consumer Health on the Internet*, **24** (3), 278–84.
https://doi.org/10.1080/15398285.2020.1791670.

Health Education England (2021) *Knowledge for Healthcare: Mobilising Evidence; Sharing Knowledge; Improving Outcomes. A Strategic Framework for NHS Knowledge and Library Services 2021–2026.*
www.hee.nhs.uk/our-work/knowledge-for-healthcare.

Lewandowsky, S., Ecker, U. K. H., Seifert, C. M., Schwarz, N. and Cook, J. (2012) Misinformation and its Correction, Continued Influence and Successful Debiasing, *Psychological Science in the Public Interest*, **13** (3),106–31. https://doi.org/10.1177/1529100612451018.

Lloyds Bank (2021) *UK Consumer Digital Index.*
www.lloydsbank.com/banking-with-us/whats-happening/consumer-digital-index.html.

McKenna, V. B., Sixsmith, J. and Barry, M. M. (2017) The Relevance of Context in Understanding Health Literacy Skills: Findings from a Qualitative Study, *Health Expectations*, **20** (5), 1049–60.
https://onlinelibrary.wiley.com/doi/full/10.1111/hex.12547.

National Academy on an Aging Society and The Center for Health Care Strategies (1999) Low Health Literacy Skills Increase Annual Health Care Expenditures by $73 Billion. In Batterham, R. W., Buchbinder, R., Beauchamp A., Dodson, S., Elsworth, G. R. and Osborne, R. H. (2014) The OPtimising HEalth LIterAcy (Ophelia) Process: Study Protocol for Using Health Literacy Profiling and Community Engagement to Create and Implement Health Reform, *BMC Public Health*, 14, 694. https://doi.org/10.1186/1471-2458-14-694.

National Institute for Health and Care Excellence (NICE) (2021) *Guideline on shared decision making.* www.nice.org.uk/guidance/ng197/chapter/Recommendations.

NHS Education for Scotland and Health Education England (2020) *eLearning for Healthcare Health Literacy Programme.* www.e-lfh.org.uk/health-literacy.

NHS England (2016) *Accessible Information Standard.* www.england.nhs.uk/ourwork/accessibleinfo.

NHS England (2023) *Health Literacy Toolkit. Second edition.* www.library.nhs.uk/health-information.

Nutbeam, D. (2000) Health Literacy as a Public Health Goal: A Challenge for Contemporary Health Education and Communication Strategies into the 21st Century, *Health Promotion International*, 15 (3), 259–67. https://doi.org/10.1093/heapro/15.3.259.

Paasche-Orlow, M. K., Parker, R. M., Gazmararian, J. A., Nielsen-Bohlman, L. T. and Rudd, R. R. (2005) The Prevalence of Limited Health Literacy, *Journal of General Internal Medicine*, 20 (2), 175–84. https://link.springer.com/content/pdf/10.1111/j.1525-1497.2005.40245.x.pdf.

Patient Information Forum (2013) *Making the Case for Information: The Evidence for Investing in High Quality Health Information for Patients and the Public.* https://pifonline.org.uk/download/file/41.

Patient UK (2022) *Metronidazole for Bacterial Infection.* https://patient.info/medicine/metronidazole-for-infection-flagyl#nav-2.

Pifalo, V., Hollander, S., Henderson, C. L., DeSalzo, P. and Gill, G. P. (1997) The Impact of Consumer Health Information Provided by Libraries: The Delaware Experience. 96th Annual Meeting of the Medical Library Association, *Bulletin of the Medical Library Association*, 85 (1), 16–22. www.ncbi.nlm.nih.gov/pmc/articles/PMC226218/pdf/mlab00094-0030.pdf.

Public Health England and UCL Institute of Health Equity (2015) *Local Action on Health Inequalities – Improving Health Literacy to Reduce Health Inequalities: Practice Resource Summary.*

www.gov.uk/government/publications/local-action-on-health-inequalities-improving-health-literacy.

Rowlands, G., Protheroe, J., Richardson, M., Ruddet, R., Seed, P. T. and Winkley, J. (2015) A Mismatch Between Population Health Literacy and the Complexity of Health Information: An Observational Study, *British Journal of General Practice*, **65** (635), e379–86.

Rudd, R. E. (2007) Health Literacy Skills of US Adults, *American Journal of Health Behavior*, **31**, S8–18. www.ingentaconnect.com/content/png/ajhb/2007/00000031/a00100s1/art 00003.

Saironen, A. and Savolainen, R. (2010) Avoiding Health Information in the Context of Uncertainty Management, *Information Research*, **15** (4). http://informationr.net/ir/15-4/paper443.html.

Shannon Trust (2022) www.shannontrust.org.uk/in-prisons.

Sorensen, K., Pelikan, J. M., Rothlin, F., Ganahl, K., Slonska, Z., Doyle, G., Fullam, J., Kondilis, B., Agrafiotis, D., Uiters, E., Falcon, M., Mensing, M., Tchamov, K., van Den Broucke, S. and Brand, H. (2015) Health Literacy in Europe: Comparative Results of the European Health Literacy Survey (HLS-EU), *The European Journal of Public Health*, **25** (6), 1053–8.

Spring, M. (2020) Coronavirus: The Human Cost of Virus Misinformation, *BBC News*, 27 May. www.bbc.co.uk/news/stories-52731624.

Sykes, S., Wills, J., Rowlands, G. and Popple, K. (2013) Understanding Critical Health Literacy: A Concept Analysis, *BMC Public Health*, **13**, 150. https://bmcpublichealth.biomedcentral.com/articles/10.1186/1471-2458.

University of Southampton (2020) *Health Literacy*. http://healthliteracy.geodata.uk.

von Wagner, C., Knight, K., Steptoe, A. and Wardle, J. (2007) Functional Health Literacy and Health-Promoting Behaviour in a National Sample of British Adults, *Journal of Epidemiology and Community Health*, **61** (12), 1086–90.

Walton, G., Barker, J., Turner, M., Pointon, M. and Wilkinson, A. (2022) Information Discernment and the Psychophysiological Effects of Misinformation, *Global Knowledge, Memory and Communication* (previously *Library Review*), **71** (8/9), 873–98. https://doi.org/10.1108/GKMC-03-2021-0052.

Wolf, M. S., Feinglass, J., Thompson, J. and Baker, D. W. (2010) In Search of 'Low Health Literacy': Threshold vs Gradient Effect of Literacy on Health Status and Mortality, *Social Science and Medicine*, **70** (9), 1335–41.

Zaracostas, J. (2020) How to Fight an Infodemic, *The Lancet*, **395** (10225), 676. www.thelancet.com/journals/lancet/article/PIIS0140-6736(20)30461-X/fulltext.

Further reading

NHS (2019) *NHS Long Term Plan.* www.longtermplan.nhs.uk.

Office for National Statistics (2021) *Health State Life Expectancies by National Deprivation Deciles, England and Wales: 2017 to 2019.* www.ons.gov.uk/peoplepopulationandcommunity/healthandsocialcare/healthinequalities.

Patient Information Forum (2014) *What Does Good Health Information Look Like?* https://pifonline.org.uk/download/file/241.

The King's Fund (2021) *Health Inequalities in a Nutshell.* https://tinyurl.com/HealthInequalitiesinanutshell.

Additional resources

Aqua: *Shared Decision Making – Ask 3 Questions Tool.* https://aqua.nhs.uk/resources/shared-decision-making-ask-3-questions.

CRAAP Test. https://researchguides.ben.edu/source-evaluation.

DISCERN. www.discern.org.uk.

European Health Literacy Survey (HLS–EU), *European Journal of Public Health*, **25** (6), 1053–8. https://doi.org/10.1093/eurpub/ckv043.

Hemingway Editor. https://hemingwayapp.com.

HM Government: *SHARE Checklist*. https://sharechecklist.gov.uk.

MacMillan Cancer Information and Support. www.macmillan.org.uk/cancer-information-and-support.

NHS Digital Service Manual: Content Style Guide. https://service-manual.nhs.uk/content.

NHS website: www.nhs.uk.

Plain English Campaign Free Guides: www.plainenglish.co.uk/freeguides.html.

Royal College of Obstetricians and Gynaecologists: *Patient Information.* www.rcog.org.uk/en/patients.

SMOG Readability Formula Tool: https://readabilityformulas.com/smogreadability-formula.php.

8

Resource Discovery and Open Access

Hélène Gorring and Fran Wilkie

Introduction

What do we mean by 'resource discovery'? Access to up-to-date information is critical for supporting day-to-day decision making in health. To deliver high quality care and support to patients, service users, carers and families, NHS staff need easy access to current and quality knowledge resources. The vision of HEE's Knowledge for Healthcare strategy is for staff, learners and the public to use the right knowledge, at the right time, in the right place to achieve excellence in healthcare.

We are talking about resources, such as books, journals and databases, as well as the infrastructure, such as library management systems, discovery systems and authentication.

As we've learned in other chapters, this is a distributed, mobile workforce comprising busy, time-poor staff: we cannot always reasonably expect them to visit physical libraries to access printed material, so e-resources are a key means to make knowledge available to the health and care workforce.

A key factor influencing resource discovery in the NHS is of course continuous advances in technology and the growing expectations of 'digitally-savvy' generations of staff and learners, to some extent countered by the limitations of information technology in the NHS and the need to support all staff, regardless of digital literacy levels.

Historically, NHS libraries were largely funded from medical education budgets and the content held within them was largely aimed at medical staff. However, libraries have become fully multi-disciplinary and now need to meet the needs not only of all types of clinical staff, but anyone that works in the organisation. As such, the resources they provide need to encompass the needs of all these staff groups as well as the students on placement within the organisation.

Open access has become a growing imperative and we conclude this chapter by defining what this means within a healthcare context and the NHS.

Types of resources

Books

Books often provide useful background or introductory information on a topic. Potentially helpful for healthcare staff at different points throughout their careers, they are particularly popular with those on education courses and students on placement in NHS organisations, who will typically have a recommended reading list from their university.

Book records are added to the catalogues of library management systems (LMS). Most NHS libraries in England now participate in regional LMS, enabling library service users to find and request books held in any library in the region, as well as reducing the library staff time involved in adding new titles.

Books will be assigned a classmark so that users can more easily find them on the shelves. There are several classification and indexing schemes in use across the NHS, but the most widely used is the Wessex Scheme (SWIMS Network, 2013), a version of the National Library of Medicine (NLM) scheme adapted to reflect UK health practice.

However, with NHS staff being geographically dispersed and unlikely to necessarily have a physical library at their site of work, e-books are ideal for this sector. The need for e-books became ever more evident through the COVID pandemic when most physical libraries closed and provided their services virtually. Unfortunately, e-books are a complex area; too often they are unaffordable for health and care library services and are inappropriately priced.

Some e-books are a PDF version of a printed text, others are in ePub format with more interactive and multimedia elements. Others are more like websites, like the British National Formulary (BNF), which has all the drug information and their contra-indications and is used by pharmacists and medical and non-medical prescribers, or the Royal Marsden Manual, a key resource for nurses.

Adding to the complexity is the fact that e-books are made available on a range of supplier platforms. Libraries can buy titles directly from book publishers (key publishers in health include BMJ, Oxford University Press and Wiley) or they can purchase them via an aggregator (examples include EBSCO, Kortext and Proquest). To effectively meet the needs of their diverse user groups, libraries must buy from more than one supplier. The fact that each uses a different platform almost inevitably makes discovery of e-books quite fragmented.

The final area of complexity surrounds purchasing models and pricing. Suppliers typically offer a range of purchasing models, including subscriptions whereby libraries pay a renewal cost each year, e-books that can be purchased 'in perpetuity' so that a library owns the title outright, as well as short loan and credit models. 'Patron driven acquisition', where available, can be useful to encourage users to recommend titles to the library for purchase. Titles may be subscribed to or purchased individually or in 'bundles'. In theory, this wide choice provides flexibility for NHS librarians trying to meet the diverse needs of their users, but in practice, pricing may mean that it is not cost-effective or even affordable to provide e-books.

These issues are not unique to the health sector and there has been a university libraries'-led 'E-book SOS' campaign, challenging publishing practices that are making e-books unaffordable and inaccessible to libraries and calling for regulation of the market (SCONUL, 2021).

Journals

Journals are a key source of information for healthcare staff to access the latest research. Some library services continue to buy print copies of a number of titles, but most journals are now bought as online only publications. This means that staff can access them from wherever they have internet access, rather than having to go to the library to find a copy.

Journals are usually published on a quarterly, monthly or weekly basis, so they feel very up to date. However, scientific articles go through a formal peer review process and the time to get to publication can take several months. Accessing preprints is a way of speeding up this process. A preprint is a version of a scientific manuscript posted on a public server before the peer review. They became increasingly important during the COVID pandemic when there was a greater need for rapid data sharing.

Journals typically include a number of different types of articles, ranging from letters and opinion pieces, to reports of individual clinical trials, to systematic reviews that try to identify all the evidence on a topic. ('Evidence' is defined in Chapter 5 on Mobilising Evidence and Knowledge.)

Many journals need a subscription to access them. Similar to e-books, there are several different ways that library services can purchase online journals. They can buy individual titles or packages of titles from different publishers or bundles of titles from subscription agents. However, there is a growing movement towards open access publishing, where articles are available free for all to read; we will come back to this at the end of this chapter.

Bibliographic databases

Bibliographic databases are organised collections of references to published papers, including journal articles, conference papers, reports, government publications and books. They contain rich metadata to identify and describe the contents of each item. They used to be published in the form of space-consuming printed indexes, then became available for libraries to buy in compact, digital disc formats. They are now produced as online resources, with interfaces designed to help users search effectively.

Databases are owned by different companies and are not usually freely available; a subscription is needed to log in and access them.

There are several bibliographic databases that cover just healthcare-related information. Some are more general in scope and some focus on specific aspects of care, such as nursing or psychology. Some of the databases overlap with each other in terms of scope and the articles they index.

Several databases are purchased for health and social care staff working in the NHS in England (see the section below 'How does funding and purchasing work in the NHS?'), with the intention of covering as wide a range of information as possible. At the time of writing, these include:

- AMED – covering allied and complementary medicine, including palliative care
- BNI – the British Nursing Index, covering nursing, midwifery and community healthcare
- CINAHL – covering nursing and allied health professions
- Embase – covering biomedical and pharmaceutical information
- Emcare – covering nursing and allied health
- HMIC – covering healthcare management information
- Medline – covering biomedical, life sciences, allied health and pre-clinical sciences information
- PsycInfo – covering psychology, behavioural sciences and related disciplines
- Social Policy and Practice – covering health and social care.

Health and care staff in England also have access to the Cochrane Library via a national contract. The Cochrane Library is a collection of databases that contain high quality evidence to inform healthcare decision-making. The core database is the Cochrane Database of Systematic Reviews, which are all produced to rigorous standards and clearly lay out the evidence with implications for practice and for further research.

A short history of database provision in the NHS in England
From 2008 to 2022, staff in the NHS in England had access to a resource called HDAS (Healthcare Databases Advanced Search). This was provided firstly by the National Library for Health and then by NICE (the National

Institute for Health and Care Excellence), to make accessing and using bibliographic databases easier. Each database provider has a different interface for its products and while the principles of searching in the databases are common, there are nuances between them: remembering which symbol to use for truncation for which, for example, made searching more difficult for people who don't use them regularly. HDAS was designed to be one search interface that could have any number of different databases plugged in behind it, so that searchers only had to learn how to use the one interface. It also allowed people to search across databases from different providers at the same time, although doing so limited the search features and functions available.

However, with the increasing complexity of the number of database providers, the decision was made to decommission HDAS at the end of March 2022. Health and care staff in England can now choose to search the individual databases if they need an in-depth search, or search for articles using the national resource discovery service (more on this below) if they prefer a simpler search. Where staff have access to a funded library service, they can also get support with searching from the knowledge and library staff in their organisations.

Why do we use journals and bibliographic databases?

Health and care staff need to find the best available evidence to answer questions about how to treat and care for patients and service users. A core principle of evidence-based medicine is that there is a hierarchy of evidence, with systematic reviews and meta-analyses that combine the results of several studies being seen as more reliable or better evidence than the results of single studies. Similarly, randomised controlled trials are seen as more reliable evidence than cohort studies or case studies (Guyatt et al., 1995, 1800–4). This evidence is published in journals. But searching through individual journals for articles is incredibly time-consuming and inefficient. Instead, bibliographic databases are used to search for articles on specific topics. Once a list of relevant papers has been identified, users would then either follow links to get full text papers from online journals (if link resolver systems are set up to do this) or use their library to get copies of the papers. We will go into more detail about link resolver systems later on.

However, it has been recognised that different types of questions need different types of evidence to answer them and not all areas of health and care research lend themselves to all types of trial or study. So, searching for evidence to answer a question (literature searching) can be a difficult task. In addition, articles need to be critically appraised to determine if the research is robust and applicable. Many health libraries will provide training on this for their users. Training might include sessions on how to search bibliographic databases or how to appraise the papers that are found.

In many academic libraries, health librarians will be heavily involved in carrying out the searches for systematic reviews. In the NHS, literature searches will generally be in response to clinical and management queries – see Figure 8.1 for an example.

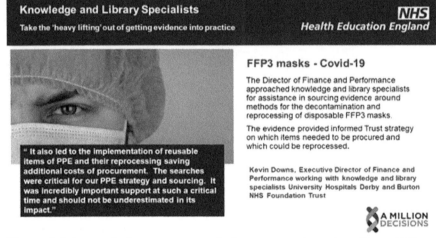

Knowledge and Library Specialists
Take the 'heavy lifting' out of getting evidence into practice

NHS
Health Education England

FFP3 masks - Covid-19

The Director of Finance and Performance approached knowledge and library specialists for assistance in sourcing evidence around methods for the decontamination and reprocessing of disposable FFP3 masks.

The evidence provided informed Trust strategy on which items needed to be procured and which could be reprocessed.

" It also led to the implementation of reusable items of PPE and their reprocessing saving additional costs of procurement. The searches were critical for our PPE strategy and sourcing. It was incredibly important support at such a critical time and should not be underestimated in its impact."

Kevin Downs, Executive Director of Finance and Performance working with knowledge and library specialists University Hospitals Derby and Burton NHS Foundation Trust

A MILLION DECISIONS

Figure 8.1 *Case study vignette – Impact of a literature search conducted by an NHS library*

In a university setting, librarians would not provide a mediated literature search service for students as it is a core part of their study to learn how to do this themselves, but in the NHS, whilst information searching skills training is a key service, the gift of time to clinicians is particularly important.

Clinical decision support tools

Sometimes referred to as 'point of care' resources, clinical decision support tools provide guidance on diagnosis, prognosis, treatment and prevention as well as medical calculators, how-to videos and patient information leaflets. They comprise synthesised research summaries and are aimed at busy clinical staff who need quick access to evidence.

There are several commercial resources on the market, such as BMJ Best Practice, Dynamed and Up to Date.

These tools can also be integrated into the Electronic Health Record systems used by NHS organisations so that the summarised evidence they provide is available to clinicians alongside patient data.

In addition to these resources, NHS staff make extensive use of guidelines and guidance produced by NICE and other organisations. These collections of evidence-based recommendations are aimed at health and social care staff, to help them make decisions about the care they're providing. NICE also commissions and funds a product called Clinical Knowledge Summaries (CKS), which are concise summaries of current evidence on the most significant and common topics in primary care.

Other resources
Other resources that health libraries might provide include:

- anatomy resources – a range of digital products are on the market around anatomy to help students understand the structure and function of the human body through multimedia images.
- exam resources – a core user group for NHS libraries are doctors in training, who will be completing exams for their specialty as they progress from medical school to Consultant grade. Books supporting these courses and revision texts are popular for this group.
- fiction, wellbeing and other general books – health libraries may also stock a range of fiction and other titles selected to support NHS staff health and wellbeing. Fiction can also be used from the angle of the medical humanities: the arts, and fictional or biographic works, can help clinicians to gain greater insight into particular conditions, illness and suffering.

Some libraries also take part in initiatives to extend their reach and attract staff who may not have previously considered using their services. Examples include the Reading Agency's '6 Book Challenge' and the opportunity to link this in with literacy work that might be taking place.

Case study 8.1 illustrates how an NHS library service runs a virtual reading group to engage users with its wider collection.

___

Case Study 8.1: Running a medical humanities book group using fiction books
Team leads: Emma Aldrich, Head of Library and Knowledge Services, and Hayley Beresford, Clinical Librarian.
Trust: Maidstone and Tunbridge Wells NHS Trust
The book club is a bi-monthly reading group that meets virtually on Twitter and Facebook to read, reflect upon and discuss questions and ideas related to medical humanities literature. The titles, chosen by our staff and social media

followers, include topics such as health, ethics, culture, disability, recovery and survivorship, wellbeing and many more. Through reading, interpretation and discussion we hope to encourage an understanding of the patient as a whole person – connected to culture and community, with their own history, experiences, emotions and values – rather than just a condition or collection of symptoms. Equally, medical humanities literature offers opportunities to practice introspection, self-analysis and empathetic concern – skills that are vital for a caring profession. As such, we see the book club as an important conduit for education, professional development, personal growth and wellbeing for our staff and followers.

Book club meetings were initially face-to-face, but the COVID-19 pandemic prompted us to think differently about how we could continue to provide a much-valued and regularly attended club when time, travel and socialising were restricted. They now run virtually using social media tools such as Twitter and Facebook.

Where possible we wanted the book club to reflect the advances in, and conversations around, health care, and science. We have done this by aligning our shortlisted titles with topical themes and recognised awareness days/weeks/months. For instance, to mark Black History Month we read *Why I'm No Longer Talking to White People About Race* by Reni Eddo-Lodge. To celebrate Health Education England and The Reading Agency's 'Uplifting Resources for NHS Staff' collection we read *Where the Crawdads Sing* by Delia Owens.

Key themes: medical humanities, reading group, wellbeing

Systems

Library management systems

In 2016, an audit of library management systems (LMS) in the NHS in England found that there were over 90 separate systems across the country. Since then, an ambitious programme has been underway to move to nationally funded, regionally shared LMS, and there is now one of these in each NHS region.

These shared systems deliver a number of benefits, including access to a greater range of resources and improved consistency for users, time savings and workflow efficiencies for library staff and cost savings for local NHS organisations. A further advantage is that it has been possible to include the catalogues of the regional LMS as search targets for the national discovery system.

LMS are critical to the day-to-day operation of library services. The implementation of each regional system has been a significant change project and the involvement of local library staff in planning and shared decision-making at every stage in selection, configuration and implementation of shared systems is critical to their success.

There are several LMS on the market and open source systems, such as Koha, which enable more customisation, are increasingly popular in health libraries.

Link resolver

Link resolver software converts bibliographic metadata into clickable web addresses. A link resolver system can therefore provide a bridge between library systems and resources, helping to provide seamless access from search tools to full text content resources. This makes it easier for users to access the content that's available to them; they can search in a bibliographic database and then, if their library has a subscription to a particular journal, click on a link to seamlessly get access to an article.

The NHS in England has a single, national link resolver system. Data relating to nationally purchased and open access journals is added nationally and local NHS libraries add data relating to their local collections. The aim is to use the link resolver to enable easy access to any resources that an individual is entitled to. The link resolver details are added to the national resource discovery system and to the nationally purchased bibliographic databases so that users get their links to full text wherever they are searching for articles.

In addition, for the NHS in England, a link enhancer service is used. This takes data from the link resolver to provide links to full text articles from other places that an end user may be searching, such as Google Scholar.

Document supply and copyright

One of the core services provided by NHS libraries is the supply of books, journal articles and other documents on request. Library staff need to make it easy for users to request items and then source and supply them as quickly as possible, in convenient formats, whilst ensuring compliance with copyright requirements.

The small size and limited holdings of NHS libraries, and the diverse and often very specific needs of their users, mean that libraries often must source items externally. There is a long history of reciprocal sharing of resources by NHS libraries, especially on a regional basis, with non-NHS healthcare libraries sometimes participating in regional resource sharing networks and the British Library and other specialist libraries typically used to source items not available within the region.

In 2018/19, around 77,000 journal articles and 42,000 books were requested by or supplied to NHS library services in England (Health Education England, 2021).

Copyright is a key consideration for library staff involved in the delivery of document supply services. Under copyright legislation, not-for-profit libraries may supply single copies of one article from a journal issue, or up to 5% of a book, on receipt of a declaration that the copy is for private study or non-commercial research and will not be shared with others. These 'library privilege' copies will not meet the needs of most healthcare library service users, who typically require copies for work purposes and need to be able to share these with others.

For this reason, the NHS in England, in common with many other organisations, including universities, local authorities and the NHS in other parts of the UK, has a licence from the Copyright Licensing Agency (CLA). The licence permits more generous sharing of copies made from journals and books that are purchased by, or subscribed to, by that organisation.

The CLA licence for the NHS in England is funded by the Department of Health and Social Care and helpfully regards the NHS in England as a single entity. This means that copyright works owned by any of the multitude of organisations that make up the NHS may be shared under the licence with any of the others within it. This thereby facilitates the extensive reciprocal interlibrary document supply that takes place between NHS libraries in England, enabling them to better support their users' needs.

Where copies required by library users cannot be sourced within the NHS in England, library staff must try to source them from external sources. Where copies are required for private study only, a library privilege copy from the British Library or another library outside the NHS in England may suffice, however, if the copy is required for sharing onwards a 'copyright fee paid' version must be obtained at additional cost, which covers the publisher.

A number of systems have been put in place and evolved over the years to help library staff manage requests and source and supply items as quickly and cost-effectively as possible, while ensuring processes are fully copyright compliant. The growth in the number of readily accessible open access journal articles, and the introduction of library discovery systems, have impacted on interlibrary document supply in different ways, whilst the huge diversity of items requested, the large range of potential sources, lack of interoperability between systems, and the inherent complexity of the NHS together mean that workflows continue to be complicated and there is always scope for further streamlining.

Development of a national discovery platform for the NHS in England

The NHS in England is made up of a large number of organisations and has more than 180 separate library services. This means that resource discovery had become highly localised. In recent years, an effort has been made to centralise activity where appropriate and provide a more cohesive and streamlined infrastructure. A pilot National electronic Library for Health (NeLH) website was launched in November 2000, which was a first attempt to bring together links to core collections of healthcare resources and specialist resources. The website went through several iterations, renamed to become the National Library for Health in 2004, then NHS Evidence in 2009, then NICE Evidence Search in 2014. A search engine was developed that allowed people to search across several resources at the same time; another first. This search function was further developed into what became known as HDAS (see the section above on bibliographic databases). The aim of the service from the start was to make it easier for health and care staff to access the best available evidence, bringing the best resources together in one place.

NICE Evidence Search and HDAS were decommissioned in March 2022, which coincided with the launch of Health Education England's new national resource discovery service (discussed below).

National discovery service in England

In 2021, Health Education England started the roll-out of a new national discovery service for the NHS in England, with the official launch in January 2022. The discovery service aims to provide NHS staff and learners with a single, coherent gateway to their trusted knowledge and library service, connecting them seamlessly to quality resources, services and support tailored to their needs. This brings together local as well as nationally purchased resources. See Figure 8.2 below for a screenshot of the search box on the homepage.

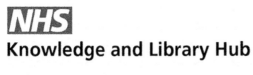

Figure 8.2 *The NHS Knowledge and Library Hub – a national discovery service in England*

Before this, the infrastructure was fragmented, with users confused about where to go for what information. The infographic in Figure 8.3 illustrates the user journey before and after the implementation.

In the **before** picture, the user has access to many resources from different places.

The **after** picture demonstrates how the national service brings lots of benefits for healthcare staff and students. There is now a single place to go to access resources, with an easy-to-use basic search. Advanced searching options are also available. Organisations have been able to personalise their version of the service, including adding links to their locally purchased resources and options to contact the library service. An extra link enhancement technology has been integrated into the service, helping users find the full text resources when they're available, with an integrated document request form for organisations with a library service. The regional LMS are also integrated, so that staff and students can access their library's book collections as well as journals and databases and other electronic resources.

Do you have a similar resource discovery system available to you? It's taken a lot of time and effort to get this one set up, involving co-ordination and co-operation between lots of different resource providers. What would be the drivers and barriers to you using a tool like this?

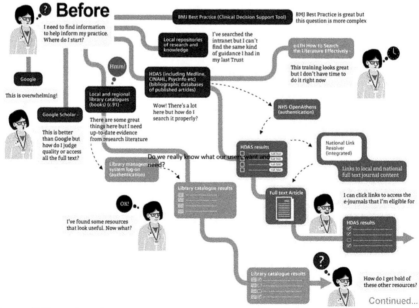

Figure 8.3 *Continued on next page*

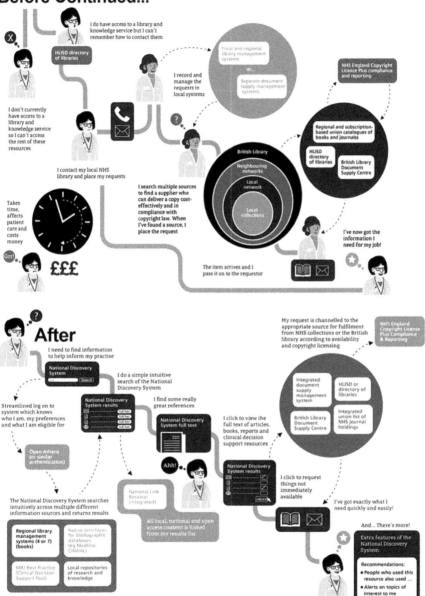

Figure 8.3 *The user journey before and after the implementation of a national discovery service in the NHS in England*

Authentication

The key to accessing all these resources seamlessly is authentication. The primary authentication system currently used across the NHS in England is OpenAthens, which is provided via a national contract with JISC. Other alternatives include IP (internet protocol) address authentication and separate usernames and passwords for individual resources. Universities use other authentication systems such as Shibboleth. Using the NHS OpenAthens authentication system means that eligible staff and students have a single username and password that they can use to access all the OpenAthens authenticated resources. Once someone logs in to one resource with their OpenAthens account, they can then move between different resources without needing to keep logging in.

The NHS OpenAthens eligibility criteria are designed to be as inclusive as possible to accommodate all those involved in the delivery of publicly funded care. The criteria have been iterated over time to reflect changes in the organisation of the NHS.

Collection development and management

How does funding and purchasing work in the NHS?

Since 2002, a set of resources (referred to as the 'national core content collection') has been purchased and made available to all healthcare staff and learners in England. However, about 75% of NHS investment in digital knowledge resources takes place at local NHS trust level. Health Education England carries out a biannual audit of local procurement and uses the results to target negotiations with suppliers. It is aiming to achieve value for money by agreeing equitable and transparent pricing structures based on workforce numbers and usage.

Public spending is tightly controlled so most of the purchasing, whether national or local, must follow formal procurement processes. To aid this, NICE has procured and maintains a framework agreement for buying books, journals and databases, which may be used by any NHS or public sector healthcare organisation in the UK. This sets out procurement principles and agreed terms and conditions for the supply of different products.

The national core content collection focuses mostly on bibliographic databases and full text journal packages. There is a formal procurement process for buying this content and contracts are usually held for three years at a time. There is always a balance to be maintained between enabling topic coverage across all of health and social care and getting the best value for money. Health Education England also buys other key content as funding allows.

Each library service will have a varying budget to spend on resources to top up and complement what is purchased nationally by the NHS.

CILIP's Health Libraries Group co-ordinates a series of guides entitled 'Core Collections in ...' covering medicine, nursing and a few other specialties. These provide health librarians with a useful guide to support acquisitions of books for their libraries.

Case Study 8.2: Collection development within an acute hospital library

Team/project lead: Steve Glover, Head of Library Services
Trust: Manchester University NHS Foundation Trust

Manchester University NHS Foundation Trust is one of the largest teaching hospitals in England with nearly 30,000 staff and students on clinical placement from higher education institutions. The Trust is also a leading member of the NHS National Institute for Health Research (NIHR) Manchester Biomedical Research Centre and has several international centres of excellence.

Providing a knowledge and library service to such a large complex organisation presents several challenges. In the NHS financial year 2023/24, 67% of the operational budget was allocated to staffing and 33% was allocated to resources and administration, of which 73% was spent on online journals.

With collection development, we're trying to provide resources for a wide range of workforce professions at different career stages and get value for money while retaining quality and breadth of coverage. Fortunately, in the NHS we benefit from the national purchasing strategy and inherit access to centrally purchased resources. This allows local NHS library services to 'top up' the core offer with collections targeted at certain staff groups or specialties. Local purchasing is guided by cost/use metrics. Other factors influencing the purchasing of bespoke content is consortia pricing models, where groups of organisations can pool purchasing budgets to achieve discounts.

Driving library patrons to the content is important to ensure the resources provided nationally and locally deliver value for money and yield a good return on investment. All routes of access should be exploited to make the content available with the easiest possible user journey.

Key themes: collections management, purchasing

Do we really know what our users want and need?

We've seen that a lot of money is spent across the NHS in England on building collections of resources. But we have to make sure that those resources and services are meeting the needs of the range of staff groups that use knowledge and library services.

Health Education England has carried out a large amount of user research to inform its national developments. A specialist user experience (UX) organisation was commissioned to undertake this work, looking at how NHS staff and learners access and use information. The standard model they used was:

- to carry out interviews with representatives of the target audience
- where possible, to carry out site visits to sit with individuals while they carry out various tasks
- to hold a workshop where representatives of the various identified personas talk through their current user journey, mapping pain points
- from all these exercises, to draw up a list of expressed user needs
- to validate these user needs through a survey, which is completed by a much larger sample of the target audience.

Open access

Open access refers to content such as research outputs in journal articles and books that is freely available for all to read and to re-use without any restrictions or access fee. The content is free because a publication fee has been paid in advance of publication or because a version is shared publicly, usually in a repository.

There are three main publication routes:

- Gold – where the final article is free to read and re-use because an article publishing charge (APC) has been paid upfront by the author or their sponsor.
- Green – where the near-final draft of an article is publicly available or the final version is available after a period in a repository.
- Bronze – where the near-final draft of an article is publicly available or the final version is available after a period on a publisher site.

Open access also refers to an advocacy movement to apply pressure to academic publishers, setting out new business models challenging the current system. Plan S is an initiative for open access publishing that was launched in September 2018. The plan is supported by a coalition of international research bodies and stipulates that scientific publications that result from research funded by public grants must be published in compliant open access journals or platforms. This involves moving from a subscription model to a 'publish and read' model. As the publishing practices transition to a new model, 'transformative agreements', also sometimes referred to as 'transitional agreements', are being put in place, with contracts with publishers for a 'publish and read' policy.

Open access is a complex area and JISC has been working with the higher education sector to negotiate transformative agreements. In the NHS, this work is still in its early stages and is led by the NHS National Institute for Health Research (NIHR), which updated its open access policy on NIHR funded research in November 2021. It is aligned to the new UK Research and Innovation (UKRI) policy on open access publishing of UKRI funded research.

Many NHS organisations now have institutional repositories, often managed and maintained by library staff. Some focus purely on scholarly research, others also include 'practitioner research' and other grey literature.

'Grey' evidence and knowledge are often as important to the NHS as formally published research, but are generally less readily discoverable. It can take the form of audits, service evaluations and quality improvement projects. A lot of research in the NHS is never formally published as unless staff have an honorary contract with a local university or are working on major research linked to grants from organisations like NIHR, they do not have the funding or time in their busy schedules to support this.

Case study 5.1 in Chapter 5 is an excellent example of librarians collaborating to set up and manage a multi-organisational repository to make research more easily discoverable.

Conclusion

At the start of the chapter we posed the question of what we mean by resource discovery. As we have seen, it encompasses a very broad range of core activity in healthcare libraries. It is the combination of content, systems and people that enables our users to find the right information at the right time to do their jobs.

In recent years progress has been made to consolidate resource discovery activity in the NHS in England where appropriate, moving from a very localised service offer to enhanced collaborative working and providing a more cohesive and streamlined infrastructure.

In the future, open access developments should further change the resource discovery landscape, and this is an exciting area to keep a watchful eye on.

References

Guyatt, G. H., Sackett, D. L., Sinclair, J. C., Hayward, R., Cook, D. J. and Cook, R. J. (1995) Users' Guides to the Medical Literature. IX. A Method for Grading Health Care Recommendations, *JAMA*, **274** (22), 1800–4.

Health Education England (2021) *NHS Library Resource Sharing: Market Review and Options Appraisal*. https://library.hee.nhs.uk/resources/inter-lending-and-document-supply/resource-sharing-market-review-and-options-appraisal.

SCONUL Position paper (2021) *E-book and E-textbook: Position Paper*. www.sconul.ac.uk/sites/default/files/documents/SCONUL%20e-book%20and%20e-textbook%20Sustainability%20Position%20paper%20October%202021.pdf.

SWIMS Network (2013) *Wessex Classification Scheme*, 5th edn, SWIMS Network. www.swimsnetwork.nhs.uk/modules/cataloguing/wessex-scheme/wessex-classification-scheme-new.

9

Growing the Evidence Base in Healthcare Knowledge and Library Services

Alison Brettle and Ruth Carlyle

Introduction

This chapter introduces evidence-based library and information practice, focusing on the importance of developing the evidence base for healthcare knowledge and library services. It highlights the importance of librarians conducting research to develop the evidence base for the profession. If the research is to grow the evidence base, the authors argue that part of the research process is the sharing of findings. The chapter covers skills both for conducting research and for librarians supporting research teams.

Introducing evidence-based library and information practice

Healthcare librarianship is central to enabling health and care professionals to provide and demonstrate evidence-based practice. Evidence-based practice, which grew out of evidence-based medicine, depends upon access to and application of evidence that is based on research, alongside clinical judgement based on experience (Greenhalgh, 1999). Building on their role in providing evidence to NHS colleagues, healthcare librarians have worked with librarians across other sectors on the development of evidence-based practice for librarianship itself.

Evidence-based library and information practice (EBLIP) is an approach to professional decision-making that grew out of the initial evidence-based medicine movement, when health librarians realised the importance of practising what they were preaching to clinicians (Koufogiannakis and Brettle, 2016a). The most recent model of EBLIP (Koufogiannakis and Brettle, 2016a) promotes an overall approach to practice that is about 'being evidence-based' (see Figure 9.1 on the next page) rather than simply using evidence in decision-making. The model acknowledges the use of research evidence, local evidence and professional knowledge (Koufogiannakis, 2011, 53) and a cyclical process involving: articulating problems or questions; assembling the evidence; assessing the evidence; agreeing a way forward; and adapting by revisiting goals and reflecting in order to evaluate what is working and what needs to change (Koufogiannakis and Brettle, 2016b).

> Being evidence based involves:
>
> • questioning our practice
> • gathering or creating the evidence (through research or evaluation)
> • using information or evidence wisely
>   – to make decisions about our practice or services
>   – to improve our practice by testing our new ideas
>   – to help others make decisions about our services (by demonstrating our value and impact)
> • using our professional skills to help others (to make their own evidence-based decisions).

Figure 9.1 *Being evidence-based*, adapted from Koufogiannakis and Brettle, 2016a

The literature on the use of evidence by healthcare librarians and knowledge specialists for their own profession suggests that there is a greater emphasis on supporting evidence-based medicine rather than developing EBLIP (Spring et al., 2014). Murphy uses the analogy of a midwife, enabling others to give birth to research rather than conducting research and publishing to contribute to the evidence base for library and information practice (Murphy, 2015).

In line with the approach to being evidence-based noted in Figure 9.1 above, this chapter considers the importance of developing the evidence base for healthcare knowledge and library services. It highlights the importance of conducting research, or creating the evidence, in order to develop the evidence base for healthcare librarianship in the future. This should also involve sharing the findings from that research through publications and presentations. Furthermore, it proposes that healthcare knowledge and library services have a role in enabling health and care practitioners to access evidence from research to make decisions for health and care practice.

The importance of growing the evidence base
Rationale for developing the evidence base
Building the evidence base for healthcare knowledge and library services is important both to current and future services. Undertaking and sharing studies that provide evidence about knowledge and library practice or services enables knowledge and library practitioners to develop their skills and to learn from techniques that have provided positive outcomes in other services. For the future, it builds evidence to demonstrate the value of services and a rationale for politicians and funders to invest in healthcare knowledge and library services.

Reviews of the literature demonstrate that the need to develop the research capacity of healthcare librarians and knowledge specialists is widely recognised (Rossall et al., 2008). The development of evidence-based practice as an approach has provided an opportunity for healthcare librarians to be involved in both identifying evidence for others to use and to develop librarianship as an evidence-based profession. In order to grasp this opportunity, there is a need for healthcare librarians and knowledge specialists both to add to the evidence base and to put evidence into practice (Eldredge, 2016).

The EBLIP model described by Koufougiannakis and Brettle (2016b) highlights differences between the evidence used by librarians in their decision-making to that used by clinicians. Evidence-based medicine privileges research designs, such as the randomised controlled trial, as the gold standard method of obtaining evidence on the effectiveness of interventions. However, such study designs may not always be appropriate or feasible in a health library setting as the research questions may be different and not lend themselves to such methods (Eldredge et al., 2016a). Some of the respondents to a survey suggested that they were not putting healthcare librarianship evidence into practice as they were concerned about the quality of available evidence, raising a need for practitioners to contribute to high quality research (Cooper, 2016). The research method chosen should therefore be relevant to the question at hand and be executed as rigorously as possible. As you will see in the course of this chapter, the evidence base is growing and you have opportunities to contribute to it. The EBLIP model proposes that evidence should be relevant, credible or trustworthy, and show strength in comparison to other available evidence, and can include research evidence, local evidence and professional expertise.

International policy drivers and approaches

The policy drivers for developing the evidence base for healthcare knowledge and library services vary internationally. The International Federation of Library Associations and Institutions (IFLA) endorses the principle that high quality knowledge and library services guarantee access to information as embodied in Article 19 of the Universal Declaration of Human Rights (IFLA, 2019). As part of its strategy to enable libraries to be high quality, IFLA acts as a hub for 'authoritative and original research and sources about the library and information landscape' (IFLA, 2019). By implication, research into libraries and information services is a valued resource. On health librarianship specifically, the health and bioscience section of IFLA collaborates with the International Congress on Medical Librarianship, which has been providing an international platform since 1953 for sharing best practice (Crawford, 1995).

The core values of the Medical Library Association in the United States include the 'advancement of health information research and evidence-based practice' (Medical Library Association, 2022a). In order to promote health information research, the Medical Library Association works with medical librarians to increase their research skills and provides opportunities for publication and conference presentations. The Medical Library Association encourages research into health librarianship through buddying schemes, small-scale grants and fellowships (Medical Library Association, 2022b).

Associations for medical or health librarians encourage research and promote publication through their research journals, notably the *Journal of the Canadian Medical Libraries Association*, the *Health Information and Libraries Journal* (the journal of the CILIP Health Libraries Group in the UK), the *Journal of Health Information and Libraries Australasia*, the *Journal of Health Information and Librarianship* (Nigeria) and the *Journal of the Medical Library Association* (US).

The Health and Care Act 2022 in the UK places a duty on regional bodies across health and care, the Integrated Care Boards, to ensure the use of evidence from research in the NHS. (NB The Act covers England; Scotland, Wales and Northern Ireland have their own legislation.) This acts as a policy lever for health librarians to promote their role in access to evidence and their support for research (Carlyle, 2022). The Knowledge for Healthcare example below demonstrates how the legislative hook is used to promote the development of the evidence base for health librarianship as part of a wider quality framework.

Example: Knowledge for Healthcare

Evidence-Based Library and Information Practice for healthcare librarians in England forms part of the strategic framework Knowledge for Healthcare (Health Education England, 2021). The legislative hook for use of evidence from research that underlies the framework was initially the Health and Social Care Act 2012, later replaced by the Health and Care Act 2022. The first Act placed a duty on the Secretary of State for Health to ensure the use of evidence from research in the NHS, a duty that was moved to regional groups of health and care organisations, the Integrated Care Boards, in 2022.

NHS knowledge and library services are encouraged within the Knowledge for Healthcare framework to provide access to high quality evidence and to improve the quality of library and knowledge services, using evidence from research evidence, innovation and good practice in line with the EBLIP model (Koufogiannakis and Brettle, 2016a) described above. As part of the Quality and Improvement Outcomes Framework, a service improvement mechanism for NHS funded knowledge and library services, library and information services are encouraged to demonstrate engagement in research. It is a maturity model, with knowledge and library services that are more closely engaged in research demonstrating a higher level of maturity (see Figure 9.2).

Outcome 5: The knowledge and library services team use and contribute to the knowledge base of the profession and relevant disciplines to develop and improve knowledge and library services.
Scope: This covers knowledge and library staff keeping up to date; reviewing the literature of the field to inform service improvement; applying evidence; adopting good practice and innovation to improve knowledge and library services; and contributing to the evidence base of the profession.

Established:
- The knowledge and library services team keep up to date with good practice, innovation and evidence obtained from research.
- Current evidence, good practice and innovations are discussed within the knowledge and library services team.

Good:
- Members of the knowledge and library services team share their experience, good practice and know-how in professional networks.
- Developments and improvements of the knowledge and library service are informed by the evidence base.

Very good:
- Members of the knowledge and library services team contribute to the knowledge base of library and information science or knowledge management.
- Members of the knowledge and library services team collaborate on conducting knowledge and library research.

Excellent:
- The knowledge and library service is supported by the organisation to be research active in the fields of library and information science and/or knowledge management.
- Formal research outcomes are published by members of the team within the knowledge and library services evidence base, e.g. peer-reviewed journals.

Figure 9.2 *Extract from* Quality and Improvement Outcomes Framework for NHS Funded Knowledge and Library Services in England (NHS England, 2022)

Fundamentally, the model encourages knowledge and library specialists to move from identifying and applying evidence, to sharing descriptive accounts of their own work and then to undertaking and publishing research. To do this, healthcare librarians need research skills.

Skills for research
The EBLIP model (Koufogiannakis and Brettle, 2016b) acknowledges that research evidence is not always available and, where this is the case, health librarians need to conduct research or evaluation to provide the evidence.

Basic skills for research and evaluation

To undertake research, health librarians need to understand some research terminology, have a basic understanding of research methods and use their everyday life skills, such as reading, listening, watching, questioning, summarising, presenting, reflecting and writing. Health librarians have a head start on many researchers as they are usually familiar with literature searching and organising and summarising results. These are an important start to the research process to set the scene for the research, provide ideas on how to go about doing the research and justify why the research is being undertaken. An important distinction to understand is the difference between research and evaluation. Research is a systematic investigation to establish facts and reach new conclusions, whilst evaluation is a study with a distinctive purpose, which often involves establishing whether a service works or meets its objectives. In practice, the skills needed for research or evaluation are very much the same.

An overview of the research process

Research begins with a research question that is answered during the course of the research and keeps the study on track. The question determines the methodology or approach to the research. Research falls into three main categories: quantitative; qualitative; or mixed methods, which combines the quantitative and qualitative approaches.

The quantitative approaches are more objective, often involving experiments, proving a hypothesis or whether something has an effect. Robson (2002) describes quantitative methods as fixed designs where the researcher sets out what they want to do in advance and how they are going to do it and then follows these procedures throughout the research. An example in health libraries would be if you wanted to know if face-to-face training was better than online training in improving search skills in nurses. You could set up an experiment where one group of nurses was given face-to-face training and a second group was given the same content but delivered online. You could then test the nurses after the training to see which worked best or whether both groups learned the same skills at the same level, in which case you would know that either method of training was effective. This approach was used with undergraduate nurses who were learning about literature searching for evidence-based practice (Brettle and Raynor, 2013).

In contrast, qualitative research aims to understand behaviour or people's perceptions and is often used to understand why something is happening or how something is perceived, for example, in relation to outreach marketing (Clark, 2021).

In health librarianship, mixed methods have often been used to understand the impact of services on their users, combining quantitative questionnaires followed by qualitative interviews to understand how the information provided by librarians has been used and the difference it has made in the NHS (Ayre et al., 2018; Divall et al., 2021).

Once you have decided your question and approach, it is important to think about your methods. You need to consider how you will collect your data, who you will collect it from, your target population sample and how you will access and choose who will be in your sample. When you are thinking about these issues, you also need to consider ethics, using a principle of doing no harm to those participants in your research. You may also need to obtain ethical approval from the organisation you work for and, depending on what you are planning, you may also need to obtain approval from an organisation such as the Health Research Authority (HRA) in the UK. Finally, it is important to ensure that your study is designed and conducted as rigorously as possible so that your results are sound and believable. This is often referred to as the validity and reliability, or credibility and trustworthiness, of the research results.

Developing research skills

Research skills and knowledge come with practice. You may have a research methods module on your library degree that will provide a basic understanding of the process, methods and design. For CILIP members, the Library and Information Research Group (LIRG) has made three introductory modules about getting started in research available (Library and Information Research Group, 2022). As part of Knowledge for Healthcare, a research toolkit of resources is available for health librarians (Health Education England, 2022). There are also a number of easy-to-read textbooks that are useful, for example Grant, Sen and Spring (2013), Robson and McCarten (2015), Pickard (2018) and many YouTube tutorials on particular research methods, techniques and terminology.

In developing your research skills, you will be building on core librarianship skills. CILIP expresses this through the Professional Knowledge and Skills Base (PKSB). The research skills section, Section 9, covers 'conducting research to further the body of knowledge about the information profession, and research to better understand how stakeholders interact with our services and profession' (CILIP, 2019) (see Figure 9.3 on the next page). Research is not only a professional skill, but also draws upon core skills in sourcing, summarising and synthesising information sources.

Research skills
1   Research process: Identifying research needs, defining research questions, conducting research using appropriate methodology, methods and sources, and reporting and disseminating findings.
2   Understanding research value: Appreciating the nature and value of research for organisations and practitioners to inform service improvement and innovation. Enabling communities to appreciate the potential value, impact and limitations of research.
3   Empirical research: Using primary qualitative, quantitative or mixed methods to conduct research, such as experiments, observations, interviews and surveys.
4   Desk research: Undertaking research, including evidence synthesis, literature analysis and methods such as content analysis and historical research.
5   Statistics and statistical analysis: Analysing statistics, interpreting and presenting results; understanding published statistical analyses.
6   Understanding research contexts: Assessing the needs of a service, organisation or client and selecting appropriate research objectives, methods and ways of presenting results.
7   Communication of research findings: Appreciating the ways in which research is communicated in order to understand research and produce high value research outputs such as reports and articles, facilitating increased impact and engagement.
8   Research ethics: Appreciating ethical norms of research and any relevant laws, regulations and guidelines, and applying them in practice.
9   Research support: Supporting and advising researchers and organisations to develop policies, data management plans, processes, systems and infrastructure involved in the management and dissemination of research, research data and research evaluation.

Figure 9.3 *Research skills – Section 9 of CILIP's PKSB* (CILIP, 2019)

The American Library Association also includes research skills as a core competency for librarians, covering knowledge of qualitative and quantitative methods, principal research findings in the field of librarianship and mechanisms to appraise research (American Library Association, 2009).

Critical appraisal to develop research skills and knowledge

Reading research studies is a good way to improve your knowledge and also helps you to design studies of your own. One starting point for developing a research project would be to find a paper on a similar topic to your research idea and examine the approach and tools that have been used. Could you do something similar? Could you adapt the tools? The methods section in a research paper should read like a recipe that you can follow step by step.

Critical appraisal of papers is another way of learning about research and research methodology and is a key feature of evidence-based practice. Critical appraisal is a process of systematically examining a piece of research to judge how well it has been undertaken and whether it is valuable and relevant in a particular context. There are many tools and guides to help with critical appraisal, particularly in the healthcare context (for example, Center for Evidence Based Management, 2022) and some specific to library and information science (for example, Glynn, 2006). One approach to reading and learning about research through critical appraisal is a journal club, where professionals choose a research paper and read and discuss the merits and limitations of the paper together. Health librarians often facilitate journal clubs for staff within their own organisation, but there are journal clubs for health librarians as well, such as the Health Information and Libraries Journal Club (Fricker and Roper, 2019).

Critical appraisal tools are centred round a structured set of questions, and using them regularly with a wide range of study designs can help build skills and confidence in using, discussing and ultimately doing research. Each issue of the EBLIP journal (University of Alberta, 2022a) contains an evidence summaries section where research papers are summarised and critically appraised on behalf of practitioners. This provides an easy introduction to the idea of reading and critiquing research. Critically appraising research and applying it to your practice contributes to the 'good' and 'very good' levels of the *Quality and Improvement Outcomes Framework* summarised in Figure 9.2 on p. 147.

Skills for supporting researchers
The role of librarians in supporting researchers
Health librarians, like their counterparts in academic and other sectors, play a key role in supporting researchers, as well as undertaking their own research. Within the PKSB in Figure 9.3 on p. 150, the competencies for supporting researchers are defined as:

> Supporting and advising researchers and organisations to develop policies, data management plans, processes, systems and infrastructure involved in the management and dissemination of research, research data and research evaluation.
>
> (CILIP, 2019)

To support researchers, health librarians and knowledge specialists need to be aware of the research processes, techniques and knowledge resources applicable to organisational and individual research interests. While the research support role does not involve setting the research question, contributions from the profession will help shape the research question, particularly through providing access to the current evidence base.

The research role of knowledge and library specialists is not limited to literature searches to inform the initial research question, but can take a range of forms throughout the research process. It is a case of applying core librarianship skills and techniques to researchers as a specific user group.

Application of librarianship skills

The core skills of librarians and information professionals can be applied to supporting researchers throughout the process (Figure 9.4). As with any project, knowledge mobilisation techniques can be applied before, during and after the research study.

Options for health librarians to support researchers
- Literature review and horizon scanning to inform creation of research bids.
- Access to grey literature, including access to reports from other research studies in institutional repositories, to inform research bids and ongoing evidence review.
- Peer assist (pre-project knowledge mobilisation).
- Literature search training for research team members.
- Support for or undertaking systematic reviews.
- Advising on conference poster development, including connections within a healthcare organisation for advice on corporate identity and design support.
- Ongoing evidence alerts and horizon scanning.
- Advice on publication options, including open access.
- Retrospect (post-project knowledge mobilisation) and creating knowledge assets from the process of conducing the research.
- Repository management for the full range of assets emerging from the research.

Figure 9.4 *Applying librarianship skills to supporting researchers*

Contributions to the research process should begin before the research topic is finalised, with health librarians as part of the team developing the research bid, in particular conducting literature reviews and horizon scanning to inform the specification (see Figure 9.4). As members of the research team, part of a health librarian's time should be funded to enable them to become embedded in the research team. They can then support the team using knowledge mobilisation methods before, during and after the study, ensuring that a full set of assets is produced on the process of the research and not just any published findings.

Core librarianship activities are of great value to research teams, but may not be immediately obvious to researchers who have not previously worked with health librarians. Notably, researchers are increasingly expected to ensure that assets from their studies, such as mid-programme reports, are held within the healthcare organisation in which the research took place. Healthcare librarians who maintain repositories for their organisations are ideally placed to hold this grey literature, as well as published assets.

Impact case studies

The impact case studies in this section reflect research support provided by health librarians in England, but will be mirrored by examples elsewhere. If you are reviewing research studies, you could consider the role played by a health librarian in the research and whether they have been acknowledged in the final paper or recognised as an author.

Case Study 9.1: Dissociation and recovery in psychosis research project (DRIP)
Team: Wotton Lawn Library
Trust: Gloucestershire Health and Care NHS Foundation Trust
Target group: Research team
A research team looking at dissociation and recovery in psychosis invited a library and information specialist to be part of their research group.

Library staff provided a series of in-depth extensive literature reviews on topics jointly decided by the project group to inform the plan for research. It is recognised that the library team has extensive knowledge and experience in this area. The literature searches were instrumental in shaping the research and were published as a separate research article.
Key themes: research skills, literature review

Case Study 9.1 demonstrates how health librarians have been involved in literature reviews that informed the research planning, leading to the full literature review being published as a work of research in its own right.

Case Study 9.2: Institutional repository/research hub
Team: Patricia Bowen Library and Knowledge Service
Trust: Chelsea and Westminster Hospital NHS Foundation Trust
Target group: Research and Development team
The knowledge and library team met an organisational need by developing an institutional repository of research published by staff. The aims of the repository are:

- to collect, preserve and archive all the Trust staff research digitally
- to showcase Trust research outputs
- to make Trust research open access
- to create exposure to the work done by the Trust staff and connect with colleagues internally and externally.

Key themes: research, institutional repository, research hub

Healthcare organisations, like academic institutions, need to be accountable for research either that they have funded or to which they have contributed through the time of clinical teams or access to patients. In this context, institutional repositories, such as in Case Study 9.2, provide a valued service on multiple levels. In this instance, the NHS organisation has also been able to use the repository to make the Trust research available via OpenAccess, increasing access within the NHS to NHS funded research and raising the profile of the organisation's research outputs.

Contributing to the evidence base

Communicating research findings is one of the key skills for research outlined in the PKSB (CILIP, 2019). Communicating or disseminating research findings enables other professionals to value, use or build on your work in their own evidence-based practice. It raises the profile of your work and potentially your library service. Sharing findings also spreads innovative ideas and approaches, reducing unnecessary duplication of effort and promoting the value of the knowledge and library profession. Indeed, if you do not plan to share the results of your research, you may question the purpose of doing the research in the first place! Many practitioners find the idea of sharing their research daunting, perhaps because they fear negative feedback along the way or they feel that their work is not good enough or important enough to shout about. Practitioners value hearing about other people's work and feedback that is given is often positive, or at worst constructive to help improve the work before publication.

A good first step to disseminating your research is to write about it more informally, perhaps using a blog or a newsletter. Newsletter editors are often on the lookout for content for their publication and will welcome a report on a piece of research or innovative practice. The CILIP Health Libraries Group publish a quarterly newsletter via a WordPress blog and provide guidance for those wishing to submit a short piece (CILIP, 2022a).

For those who enjoy presenting, a conference paper or poster is an alternative way of disseminating your work. Conferences have been a little disrupted since the COVID pandemic, but many have moved online or are starting to return face-to-face. The UK CILIP Health Libraries Group holds conferences (CILIP, 2022b) and the European Association for Health Information and Libraries (EAHIL) holds an annual conference (EAHIL, 2022). Conference organisers publicise their conferences well in advance and often request submissions for presentations or posters. Producing a piece of work to a conference deadline can often be used as a motivating tool to ensure you complete the research in good time. As well as providing a great way of disseminating your own work, conferences are an excellent way of hearing about other people's work, which helps to spark new ideas and collaborations for future developments.

Local events in your workplace or in your library region are great places to communicate about the work you have been doing. Presentations are also an excellent way of gaining feedback about your work that could be incorporated into a short report or article that you publish in written form at a later date.

Traditionally, academic research is published in an academic journal. Papers submitted to academic journals will go through a peer review process, which provides feedback and aims to ensure the quality of research published. Publication in an academic journal provides recognition for your work, contributes to scholarly literature and, depending on your chosen career path, can be important for your CV. Academic journals aimed at health librarians include the *Health Information and Libraries Journal* (Wiley Online Library, 2022) and the *Journal of the Medical Library Association* (Pitt Open Library Publishing, 2022).

Writing for an academic journal can be both rewarding and challenging and requires a certain degree of writing skills (Zach, 2022). Journals that welcome articles from library practitioners who are first-time authors include the *EBLIP Journal* (University of Alberta, 2022a) and the *Library and Information Research Journal* (University of Alberta, 2022b). All these journals have sections for short reports that are not subject to a full peer review and are often a quicker and less daunting alternative to publishing your work. Publishing your work in this way would contribute to the 'very good' and 'excellent' levels of the *Quality and Improvement Outcomes Framework* described in Figure 9.2 on p. 147.

Conclusion

Increasing the evidence base for health librarianship is dependent on health librarians and knowledge specialists undertaking and publishing research. The role that health librarians play in supporting researchers provides them with insights into the research process and how health librarians can conduct research into health librarianship.

Although it is recognised that there is much more work to do, there are some areas of health librarianship where the research evidence is steadily growing and improving following systematic reviews that highlighted where research was needed. For example, Winning and Beverley (2003), Wagner and Byrd (2004) and Brettle et al. (2011) demonstrated satisfaction with clinical librarian services, but a lack of evidence on effectiveness. This led to research in the UK (Brettle, Maden and Payne, 2016; Divall et al., 2021) demonstrating the contribution of clinical librarians to patient care, continuing professional development and research, as well as a return on investment (Hartfiel et al., 2021). Put together, research, largely undertaken by health librarians, has shown that clinical librarians contribute 'a gift of time' to the NHS (Economics by Design, 2020).

Similarly, systematic reviews highlighted deficits in the evidence around training clinicians to search for evidence (Brettle, 2003; 2007; Garg and Turtle, 2003) and subsequent research used more rigorous research methods to demonstrate the effectiveness of providing training to clinicians (Gardois et al., 2011; Brettle and Raynor, 2013; Ayre et al., 2015; Eldredge, 2016b). Health librarians involved in systematic review provision have been researching this field since the 1990s (for example, Haynes et al., 1994) and are continuously adding to the evidence base around systematic searching in relation to search filters, topic searching and optimal resources for searching (Brettle, 2019; Golder et al., 2022).

Finally, there is a growing body of evidence on the impact of health librarians on patient care (largely following provision of literature search services) including Bartlett and Marshall (2013) and Marshall et al. (2014a and 2014b). Within the UK, this evidence highlighted the wider contribution of health library services to the organisation as a whole (Brettle, Maden and Payne, 2016; Ayre et al., 2018), with the development of a valid and reliable tool (Urquhart and Brettle, 2022) that can be used across any health library to provide ongoing evidence of the impact of their services.

Growing the evidence base is important to 'sustain the profession's reputation for knowledge discovery and innovation; to demonstrate professional value and impact; and, by means of its scholarly approach, to raise the profile of library and information science (LIS) as a discipline' (Pickton, 2016). By playing their role in this, health librarians are better able to develop the impact of knowledge and library services, increasing evidence use for high quality healthcare. This is a role to which you can contribute.

Reflection points
- How do you view your role in supporting researchers?
- How do you view your role in undertaking your own research?
- What areas of evidence-based library and information practice could you explore in more detail?
- What support do you need to implement evidence-based library and information practice?
- How would you present the rationale for developing the evidence base for library and information practice?
- Reflect on the distinction between:

– the skills needed as a knowledge and library practitioner to support researchers; and

– the skills needed to undertake research to increase the evidence base for library and information practice.

References

American Library Association (2009) *Final Core Competencies Statement.* www.ala.org/educationcareers/careers/corecomp/corecompetences.

Ayre, S., Brettle, A. and Gilroy, D. et al. (2018) Developing a Generic Tool to Routinely Measure the Impact of Health Libraries, *Health Information and Libraries Journal*, **35** (3), 227–45. https://doi.org/10.1111/hir.12223.

Bartlett, J. C. and Marshall, J. G. (2013) The Value of Library and Information Services in Patient Care: Canadian Results from an International Multisite Study, *Journal of the Canadian Health Libraries Association (JCHLA)*, **34** (3), 138–46. https://doi.org/10.3163%2F1536-5050.101.1.007.

Brettle, A. (2003) Information Skills Training: A Systematic Review of The Literature, *Health Information and Libraries Journal*, **20** (Suppl. 1), 3–9. https://doi.org/10.1111/j.1471-1842.2007.00740.x.

Brettle, A. (2007) Evaluating Information Skills Training in Health Libraries: A Systematic Review, *Health Information and Libraries Journal*, **24** (Suppl. 1), 18–37. https://doi.org/10.1111/j.1471-1842.2007.00740.x.

Brettle, A. (2019) The Information Specialist as an Expert Searcher. In Levay, P. and Craven, J. (eds), *Systematic Searching: Practical Ideas for Improving Results*, Facet Publishing.

Brettle, A., Maden, M. and Payne, C. (2016) The Impact of Clinical Librarian Services on Patients and Health Care Organisations, *Health Information and Libraries Journal*, **33** (2), 100–20. https://doi.org/10.1111/hir.12136.

Brettle, A., Maden-Jenkins, M., Anderson, L., McNally, R., Pratchett, T., Tancock, J., Thornton, D. and Webb, A. (2011) Evaluating Clinical Librarian Services: A Systematic Review, *Health Information and Libraries Journal*, **28** (1), 2–32.

Brettle, A. and Raynor, M. (2013) Developing Information Literacy Skills in Pre-Registration Nurses: An Experimental Study of Teaching Methods, *Nurse Education Today*, **33** (2),103–9.

Carlyle, R. (2022) Making the Most of Public Policy in Health Libraries and Information Services: Example of the Health and Care Bill 2022, *Health Information and Libraries Journal*, **39** (2), 99–101. https://doi.org/10.1111/hir.12432.

Center for Evidence Based Management (2022) *Critical Appraisal.* https://cebma.org/resources-and-tools/what-is-critical-appraisal.

Chartered Institute of Library and Information Professionals (CILIP) (2019) *The Professional Knowledge and Skills Base Assessment Tool: Developing Skills for Success*. www.cilip.org.uk/page/PKSB.

Chartered Institute of Library and Information Professionals [CILIP] (2022a) Health libraries Group Newsletter. www.cilip.org.uk/members/group_content_view.asp?group=200697&id=6 87365.

Chartered Institute of Library and Information Professionals (CILIP) (2022b) *Health Libraries Group Events/Conferences*. www.cilip.org.uk/members/group_content_view.asp?group=200697&id=6 86219.

Clark, H. (2021) Outreach Marketing may be a Successful Strategy for NHS Libraries, *Health Information and Libraries Journal*, **38** (1), 61–5. https://doi.org/10.1111/hir.12357.

Cooper, I. D. (2016) Let's Get a Stronger Evidence Base for Our Decisions, *Journal of the Medical Library Association*, **104** (4), 259–61. https://doi.org/10.5195/jmla.2016.144.

Crawford, S. Y. (1995) *The International Congress on Medical Librarianship, 1953–1995: Aims and Achievements*. Archives of the International Congress on Medical Librarianship. www.icml.org/archives/crawf.htm.

Divall, P., James, C., Heaton, M. and Brettle, A. J. (2021) UK Survey Demonstrates a Wide Range of Impacts Attributable to Clinical Librarian Services, *Health Information and Libraries Journal*, **39** (2), 116–31. https://doi.org/10.1111/hir.12389.

Economics by Design (2020) *NHS Funded Library and Knowledge Services in England – Value Proposition: The Gift of Time*. www.hee.nhs.uk/our-work/library-knowledge-services/value-proposition-gift-time.

Eldredge, J. D. (2016) Integrating Evidence into Practice, *Journal of the Medical Library Association*, **104** (4), 333–7. https://doi.org/10.5195/jmla.2016.153.

Eldredge, J. D., Gard Marshall, J., Brettle, A., Holmes, H., Haglund, L. and Wallace, R. (2016a) Health Librarians. In Koufogiannakis, D. and Brettle, A. (eds), *Being Evidence Based in Library and Information Practice*, Facet Publishing.

Eldredge, J. D., Hall, L. J., McElfresh, K. R., Warner, T. D., Stromberg, T. L., Trost, J. and Jelinek, D. A. (2016b) Rural Providers' Access to Online Resources: A Randomized Controlled Trial, *Journal of the Medical Library Association*, **104** (1), 1–9.

European Association for Health Information and Libraries (2022) *Events*. http://eahil.eu/events.

Fricker, A. and Roper, T. (2019) An Open Invitation to Join *HILJ [Journal] Club*, *Health Information and Libraries Journal*, **36** (4), 295–8. https://doi.org/10.1111/hir.12288.

Gardois, P., Calabreset, R., Columbi, N., Deplano, A. M., Lingua, C., Longo, F., Villanacci, M. C., Miniero, R. and Piga, A. (2011) Effectiveness of Bibliographic Searches Performed by Pediatric Residents and Interns Assisted by Librarians. A Randomized Controlled Trial, *Health Information and Libraries Journal*, **28** (4), 273–84.

Garg, A. and Turtle, K. M. (2003) Effectiveness of Training Health Professionals in Literature Search Skills Using Electronic Health Databases – A Critical Appraisal, *Health Information and Libraries Journal*, **20** (1), 33–4. https://doi.org/10.1046/j.1471-1842.2003.00416.x.

Glynn, L. (2006) A Critical Appraisal Tool for Library and Information Research, *Library Hi Tech*, **24** (3), 387–9. https://doi.org/10.1108/07378830610692154.

Golder, S., Farrah, K., Mierzwinski-Urban, M., Barker, B. and Rama, A. (2022) Updated Generic Search Filters for Finding Studies of Adverse Drug Effects in Ovid MEDLINE and Embase May Retrieve up to 90% of Relevant Studies, *Health Information and Libraries Journal*, 1–11. https://doi.org/10.1111/hir.12441.

Grant, M., Sen, B. and Spring, H. (eds) (2013) *Research, Evaluation and Audit*, Facet Publishing.

Greenhalgh, T. (1999) Narrative Based Medicine in an Evidence Based World, *British Medical Journal*, **318**, 323. https://doi.org/10.1136/bmj.318.7179.323.

Hartfiel N., Sadera G., Treadway V., Lawrence C. and Tudor Edwards, R. (2021) A Clinical Librarian in a Hospital Critical Care Unit May Generate a Positive Return on Investment, *Health Information and Libraries Journal*, **38** (2), 97–112. https://doi.org/10.1111/hir.12332.

Haynes, R. B., Wilczynski, N., McKibbon, K. A., Walker, C. J. and Sinclair, J. C. (1994) Developing Optimal Search Strategies for Detecting Clinically Sound Studies in MEDLINE, *Journal of the American Medical Informatics Association*, **1** (6), 447–58.

Health Education England (2021) *Knowledge for Healthcare: Mobilising Evidence; Sharing Knowledge; Improving Outcomes. A Strategic Framework for NHS Knowledge and Library Services 2021–2026*. www.hee.nhs.uk/our-work/knowledge-for-healthcare.

International Federation of Library Associations and Institutions (2019) *IFLA Strategy 2019–24*. www.ifla.org.

Koufogiannakis, D. (2011) Considering the Place of Practice-Based Evidence Within Evidence Based Library and Information Practice (EBLIP), *Library and Information Research*, **35** (111), 41–58, https://lirgjournal.org.uk/index.php/lir/article/view/486.

Koufogiannakis, D. and Brettle, A. (2016a) Introduction. In Koufogiannakis, D. and Brettle, A. (eds), *Being Evidence Based in Library and Information Practice*, 3–10, Facet Publishing.

Koufogiannakis, D. and Brettle, A. (2016b) A New Framework for EBLIP. In Koufogiannakis, D. and Brettle, A. (eds), *Being Evidence Based in Library and Information Practice*, 11–18, Facet Publishing.

Library Information and Research Group (2022) *Research eLearning*. www.cilip.org.uk/page/elearninghub.

Marshall, J. G., Sollenberger, J., Easterby-Gannett, S., Morgan, L. K., Klem, M. L., Cavanaugh, S. K., Burr Oliver, C., Thompson, C. A., Romanosky, N. and Hunter, S. (2013) The Value of Library and Information Services in Patient Care: Results of a Multisite Study, *Journal of the Medical Library Association*, **101** (1), 38–46. https://doi.org/10.3163%2F1536-5050.101.1.007.

Marshall, J. G., Morgan, J. C., Thompson, C. A. and Wells, A. L. (2014a) The Impact of Library and Information Services on Patient Quality, *International Journal of Health Care Quality Assurance*, **27** (8), 672–83.

Marshall, J. G., Morgan, J. C., Klem, M. L., Thompson, C. A. and Wells, A. L. (2014b) The Value of Library and Information Services in Nursing and Patient Care, *OJIN: Online Journal of Issues in Nursing*, **19** (3), 8. http://dx.doi.org/10.3912/OJIN.Vol19No03PPT02.

Medical Library Association (2022a) *Core Values*. www.mlanet.org.

Medical Library Association (2022b) *MLA Section Sponsored Awards and Grants*. www.mlanet.org/p/cm/ld/fid=813.

Murphy, J. (2015) Engaging in Research: Challenges and Opportunities for Health Library and Information Professionals, *Health Information and Libraries Journal*, **34** (4), 296–9. https://doi.org/10.1111/hir.12107.

Pickard, A. (2018) *Research Methods in Information*, Facet Publishing.

Pickton, M. (2016) Facilitating a Research Culture in an Academic Library: Top Down and Bottom Up Approaches, *New Library World*, **117** (1/2), 105–27. https://doi.org/10.1108/NLW-10-2015-0075.

Pitt Open Library Publishing (2022) *Journal of the Medical Library Association (JMLA)*. https://jmla.mlanet.org/ojs/jmla.

Robson, C. (2002) *Real World Research*, 2nd edn, Blackwell Publishing.

Robson, C. and McCarten, K. (2015) *Real World Research*, 4th edn, Wiley.

Rossall, H., Boyes, C., Montacute, K. and Doherty, P. (2008) Developing Research Capacity in Research: A Review of the Evidence, *Health Information and Libraries Journal*, **25** (3), 159–74. https://doi.org/10.1111/j.1471-1842.2008.00788.x.

Spring, H., Doherty, P., Boyes, C. and Wilshaw, K. (2014) Research Engagement in Health Librarianship: Outcomes of a Focus Group, *Library and Information Science Research*, **36** (3–4), 142–53. https://doi.org/10.1016/j.lisr.2014.06.004.

University of Alberta (2022a) *Evidence Based Library and Information Practice*. https://journals.library.ualberta.ca/eblip/index.php/EBLIP.

University of Alberta (2022b) *LIR Library and Information Research*. https://lirgjournal.org.uk/index.php/lir.

Urquhart, C. J. and Brettle, A. J. (2022) Validation of a Generic Impact Survey for Use by Health Library Services Indicates the Reliability of the Questionnaire, *Health Information and Libraries Journal*, **39** (4), 1–13. https://doi.org/10.1111/hir.12427.

Wagner, K. C. and Byrd, G. D. (2004) Evaluating the Effectiveness of Clinical Medical Library Programs: A Systematic Review of the Literature, *Journal of the Medical Library Association*, **92** (1), 14–33.

Wiley Online Library (2022) *Health Information and Libraries Journal*. https://onlinelibrary.wiley.com/journal/14711842.

Winning, M. A. and Beverley, C. A. (2003) Clinical Librarianship: A Systematic Review of the Literature, *Health Information Library Journal*, **20** (Suppl. 1), 10–21.

Zach, L. (2022) Writing About Research: The Good, the Bad, and the Challenging, *Evidence Based Library and Information Practice*, **17** (1), 3–4. https://doi.org/10.18438/eblip30098.

10

Measuring Progress, Value and Impact in NHS Knowledge and Library Services

Clare Edwards, Dominic Gilroy and Victoria Treadway

Introduction

Gann and Pratt (2013) observes the need for knowledge and library services to identify ways to evaluate themselves and ensure current measures have meaning for those outside the library world and in the context of an organisation's mission and objectives.

Strategic direction is important for library services. Strategy outlines the aims, vision and intentions of the service, providing an outline of work to be undertaken. For stakeholders, customers and others outside the library team, the strategy provides a reference point to understand what the library service is aiming to achieve and assures senior colleagues that the library's goals are aligned to and support those of the wider organisation. The strategy also serves as a reminder for those working in the service of high level goals, which can easily be forgotten due to the focus on day-to-day operational tasks.

However, there is a danger that strategies can become 'shelf-ware' – documents that are produced every few years but which have little day-to-day influence on the library service. To help ensure that the strategy becomes a reality, it is important to establish processes that turn these strategic plans into actions. This can be achieved with implementation plans with SMART targets (Specific, Measurable, Achievable, Realistic and Relevant, Time Bound) (see also Chapter 2). High level strategic plans can be broken down into more manageable objectives, each with specific actions attached, against which progress can be more easily tracked.

Health Education England's national Knowledge for Healthcare strategy was first launched in 2014 (Health Education England, 2014) and refreshed in 2021 (Health Education England, 2021a). The strategy was implemented using workstreams and task and finish groups made up of both the Health Education England knowledge and library team and volunteers from healthcare knowledge and library services in England. A range of measures and frameworks were employed to monitor progress against the aims and objectives within the strategy.

This chapter outlines Health Education England's and healthcare library partners' approaches to measuring progress, value and impact in relation to the development and improvement of knowledge and library services in England.

Metrics

As with all situations where organisations and services have aims and objectives, or goals they are trying to achieve, it is important to have some means of monitoring progress towards attaining those goals. This enables services to celebrate success where objectives have been achieved and to renew efforts and try different approaches where progress is slower. In the context of knowledge and library services, the aim could be to implement a strategy or to achieve a specific goal, such as increasing usage of a resource.

When Health Education England launched the Knowledge for Healthcare strategy (Health Education England, 2014) the importance of measuring progress was clear and a task and finish group of knowledge and library specialists was established to address this concern. The group carried out an extensive review to investigate what makes a good metric and examined how metrics have been used in NHS knowledge and library services. The methodology included a survey with NHS knowledge and library staff about current approaches; a review of the history of metrics in NHS libraries; and a scoping literature search.

The resulting *Principles for Metrics Report and Recommendations* (Health Education England, 2016a) identifies a set of principles for good metrics for healthcare knowledge and library services (Figure 10.1 opposite). It defines a metric as 'criteria against which something is measured' (Showers, 2015) and 'a criterion or set of criteria stated in quantifiable terms' (Oxford University Press, 2022). A simple template has been created to support development of metrics based on the principles (Figure 10.2).

Fricker (2017) emphasises how good metrics contribute to better engagement and understanding with stakeholders and highlights the principles that will equip librarians to develop meaningful metrics in support of their service development and improvement.

It is important to be aware of the limitations of metrics and avoid over reliance on figures to measure performance. Muller (2019) notes that organisations can become obsessed with metrics and warns that this can be counterproductive. Nevertheless, the sensible use of metrics as part of a wider toolkit can help knowledge and library services in their efforts to continually develop and improve.

✓	**Meaningful** - does the metric relate to the goals of the organisation, to the needs of the users and is it re-examined over time for continuing appropriateness? Do other people care about it? Combining two facets can strengthen a metric – for example usage by a particular staff group.
✓	**Actionable** – is the metric in areas which Knowledge and Library Services (KLS) can influence? Does it drive a change in behaviour? The reasons for changes to a metric should be investigated not assumed. Beware of self-imposed targets – are they meaningful to stakeholders?
✓	**Reproducible** – the metric is a piece of research so should be clearly defined in advance of use and transparent. It should be able to be replicated over time and constructed with the most robust data available. Collection of data for the metric should not be burdensome to allow repetition when required.
✓	**Comparable** – the metric can be used to see change in the KLS over time. Be cautious if trying to benchmark externally. The diversity of services must be respected – no one metric fits all.

Figure 10.1 *Metrics principles checklist*

Metric Definition:
Give your metric a brief descriptive title. Try and explain it in a couple of lines.

Why is it important?
How does it relate to strategies and business plans for the Knowledge and Library Service, Trust or NHS England? How might it relate to the Quality and Improvement Outcomes? Who is the audience?

Process for compiling the Metric:
Where does your data come from? Describe any limits or parameters applied to standard data sets. Include a link to any survey tools if applicable / possible. How often do you repeat the process? How would someone else go about repeating your metric?

What does it mean?	Desired outcomes:
How do you interpret this metric?	What would improvement look like? Do you have a level you are required to reach or aiming for in a period? You might consider what would be Red, Amber, Green scores for a dashboard.

Improvement plans:
How do you plan to make a difference to this metric in a defined period?

Reporting:
Where and how do you plan to share the metric? Is it part of a dashboard or regular service monitoring report? You could embed a sample graph.

Figure 10.2 *Quality metrics template*

Health knowledge and library service statistics

There is a long history of library professionals monitoring and using statistics in service management.

> As long as there have been libraries, there have been library statistics. It is a powerful tool in our quest to both prove our value and improve our services.
>
> (Killick, 2021, 1)

Health libraries are no exception to this and many collect a wide range of statistics at local level to monitor and inform service performance and development. In addition to the collection of data for local use, NHS health libraries in England are requested to participate in an annual data collection exercise led by Health Education England. In fact, this exercise has been conducted for over 20 years, with the information used to inform regional and national decision-making. The return rate is usually very high due to the statistics return being mandated as part of the Education Contract that NHS organisations hold with Health Education England. Specifically, the statistics collected nationally from NHS knowledge and library services fall into two categories: staffing and activity. Staffing statistics record the numbers of staff within the service, with details such as pay bands, full/part time status, qualifications and vacancy levels. Activity statistics monitor areas such as types of service users, income and expenditure, together with the numbers of loans, document supply, literature or evidence searches, and information skills training.

There are a wide variety of statistics that could be collected in relation to libraries at local or national level. A key guiding principle should be to consider what use statistics might be put to. There is little use in putting effort into collecting statistics if the resulting data is not going to be used for anything. As part of a Health Education England leadership programme project a group of NHS knowledge and library service managers researched and created a statistics toolkit (Health Education England, 2017) to provide guidance on getting the most out of the statistical data collected. Through this and other regular ongoing reflection, Health Education England has reviewed its collection exercise to ensure the data collected has a use within the national workstreams. Furthermore, over time, the statistical and other details collected from services have changed to reflect the wider library environment and strategic direction. For example, as the importance of embedded librarians (often referred to as clinical librarians in the health sector) has been recognised, a new statistic was introduced asking services to estimate the proportion of time spent delivering outreach and embedded services.

Statistics collected at national level are used by Health Education England to monitor trends and activity levels within NHS knowledge and library services and to inform policy recommendations, funding decisions and to prioritise actions, as well as assisting in monitoring progress against Knowledge for Healthcare's strategic goals, many of which are implemented at local level. In the following section, two case studies are presented to provide an illustration of how NHS knowledge and library statistics have been utilised in the work of Health Education England.

Case Study 10.1: Staff ratio recommendations

Health Education England provides funding for NHS knowledge and library services through the Education Contract it holds with NHS trusts. There is an expectation that this funding is matched by the organisation to reflect the role of the knowledge and library service beyond education. These funding arrangements have evolved inequitably across the NHS in England with the origins often lost in history. As a result, the funding available, and therefore knowledge and library staff levels, within any single NHS knowledge and library service often follows no logical pattern. There was a perceived need for a benchmark or standard against which staffing could be measured.

Health Education England was able to make use of the data collected through the annual statistics process to identify that the average staff ratio for NHS knowledge and library services in England was one qualified knowledge and library specialist for every 1,730 healthcare staff. Cross referencing to knowledge and library services in organisations that performed well in the Care Quality Commission (CQC) inspections suggested that an increased number of knowledge specialists to healthcare staff would increase the ability of this staff group to better serve the evidence needs of the organisation.

In 2020, Health Education England settled on a policy recommendation of one qualified knowledge specialist for every 1,250 healthcare staff and encouraged NHS organisations to work towards this staff ratio if they had not already achieved it (Health Education England, 2020). The business-critical benefits of embedded roles for any additional knowledge specialists recruited was also a key feature of the recommendations.

The staff ratio recommendations have been valued within many NHS knowledge and library services, with organisations making use of them to focus on building the knowledge specialist workforce. Some knowledge and library managers have already been successful in using the recommendations to develop new embedded roles within their organisations.

Health Education England's knowledge and library staff ratio recommendations helped raise awareness of the value of embedded roles leading to two-year funding for a clinical librarian post within the Radiotherapy Education Team at the Christie.

(Daniel Livesey, Library and Knowledge Service Manager, The Christie NHS Foundation Trust)

Case Study 10.2: Workforce profiling

Combined with additional data collected through our biennial workforce survey, and through other routes, the annual staffing statistics collection allows Health Education England to monitor the workforce profile. Awareness of the numbers and roles of staff working within NHS knowledge and library services informs decision-making, leading to better decisions around continuing professional development offers and other workforce interventions (Figures 10.3 and 10.4 below and opposite).

An example of this is in late 2021 when members of the national team were noticing that knowledge and library service managers were having an increasing level of difficulty recruiting to posts. It was possible to consult with staffing statistics to confirm that the trends suggest a higher level of vacancies than normal. This was confirmed through a survey of library managers, which prompted additional efforts from Health Education England aimed at tackling this challenge.

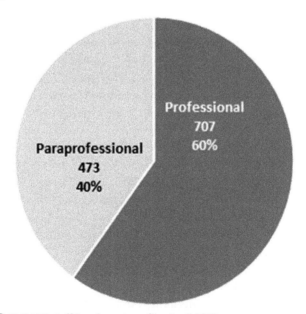

Figure 10.3 *NHS KLS staff headcount profile, April 2022*

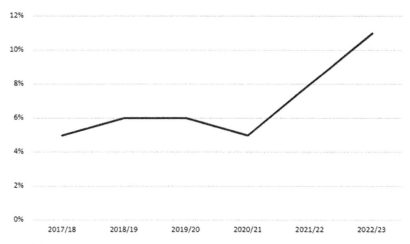

Figure 10.4 *Reported vacancy levels in NHS knowledge and library services*

Reporting on national NHS knowledge and library statistics

In addition to being useful at national level to inform decision-making and awareness, NHS knowledge and library statistics are also useful to service managers at a local level. In the early years of NHS library statistical data collection, a summary of the results was made publicly available through Loughborough University for review by interested parties (Loughborough, 2001). In more recent years, Health Education England has published infographics detailing key information relating to the statistics collected from services (Health Education England, 2021b).

Over the years, there have also been requests from library service managers who are interested in benchmarking in specific areas. For example, they may wish to know how the number of evidence searches undertaken by their service's library staff compares to the local or national average. These queries can be time-consuming to resolve and depend on the local library manager being aware that they are able to request these details from Health Education England. To streamline this process and enhance the accessibility for all managers, Health Education England is working to develop a dashboard whereby local managers are able to log in securely and compare their own service's statistical data against the country or region.

Knowledge for Healthcare Evaluation Framework

Health Education England created an impact Evaluation Framework (Health Education England, 2021c) to measure the progress of delivery of the

Knowledge for Healthcare vision. In progressing these efforts, the team worked with Sharon Markless, internationally recognised author on the topic of impact evaluation in libraries and independent impact consultant to the Bill and Melinda Gates Foundation's Global Libraries Initiative.

The Evaluation Framework was designed to provide a coherent approach to evaluating impact. It is based on the recognition that it is difficult to provide clear evidence of impact in complex systems such as healthcare. For example, it would be unrealistic to claim that the knowledge and library service, and its staff, are solely responsible for a particular positive outcome or impact. Nevertheless, it would not be unrealistic to claim that the knowledge and library service had an important role to play in the end goal being achieved.

The framework used the impact planning assessment (IPA) methodology (Streatfield 2012), which defines impact as 'any effect of the service [or of an event or initiative] on an individual or group' that aligns well with the definition in the Value and Impact Toolkit. The approach taken by IPA is to identify a series of indicators that, when taken together, suggest progress is being made. The overall emphasis in any evaluation framework is on achieving outcomes that show 'changes in behaviour, relationships, activities or actions of people, groups and organisations with whom a programme works directly' (Earl, Carden and Smutylo, 2001, 13). In the case of Knowledge for Healthcare, the working group identified a series of impact objectives representing the various workstreams within the overall strategic work programme. In total, six impact objectives were identified, each offering a succinct but clear summary statement of what will be achieved and what will be different if delivery of the vision of Knowledge for Healthcare is successful. The resulting impact objectives were as follows:

1 Health organisations mobilise evidence and internally generated knowledge to enable evidence-based policy and practice.
2 The healthcare workforce and learners receive high quality knowledge and library services.
3 Staff, learners, patients and the public are equipped to use evidence-based patient, health and wellbeing information for shared decision-making and self-care.
4 NHS funded knowledge and library services are equitable, efficient and productive.
5 The knowledge and library services workforce has the capability, confidence and capacity to meet the evolving knowledge and information needs of the healthcare system.

6   Partnership working is the norm in delivering knowledge to the
    healthcare system.

It was important to ensure that appropriate data and evidence were available
to demonstrate progress against the objectives. Since Knowledge for
Healthcare is a national strategy but is implemented largely at local level,
most of the data and evidence required is from the activity carried out by
local NHS knowledge and library services, with additional evidence from
national activity. Consequently, a monitoring dashboard was being developed
to review and report against agreed metrics and to demonstrate trends and
differences made against each of the objectives. Additionally, a review was
undertaken of the data collected from local services, and monitored at
national level, to ensure all the required areas for the Evaluation Framework
had been met.

Development of the Value and Impact Toolkit

The concept of impact is becoming increasingly important in health
knowledge and library services. What is meant by impact in the context of a
library service and why is it so important? NHS knowledge and library
services have adopted the following definition for impact:

> The difference or change in an individual or group resulting from the contact
> with library services.
>
> (International Organization for Standardization (ISO), 2014)

Impact goes beyond simple user feedback about how well a service is
performing. It is not about operational statistics, the number of evidence
searches undertaken or the number of individuals undergoing library training.
Rather, it is about the positive changes brought about by the intervention of
knowledge and library staff. Those changes may be personal to the library
patron, for example, improved knowledge or awareness, or time saved, as
demonstrated by *The Gift of Time* report (Economics by Design, 2020).
Sometimes, the changes may be much higher level, affecting entire teams,
patient groups, the organisation or the wider organisation. Examples in the
healthcare context would be where the evidence from a literature search is
used to inform changes in clinical processes and procedures, which go on to
improve patient care and lead to increased efficiency and effectiveness.

   There are many reasons why the demonstration of impact is important in
healthcare knowledge and library services. One reason is the need to ensure
that decision-making across the NHS is evidence-based wherever possible.
This is the essence of the #AMillionDecisions campaign run by CILIP's

Health Libraries Group in partnership with Health Education England. The campaign calls for decisions in the healthcare sector to be fully evidence-based, calling on government and health service providers to employ and make use of the skills of librarians and knowledge specialists in meeting their obligations under The Health and Social Care Act 2012 and its successor, The Health and Care Bill 2022. In some NHS organisations, the library service is still seen by many stakeholders as a service for students, doctors in training and those undertaking further studies. The use of impact evidence to demonstrate the far wider contribution of NHS knowledge and library services as business-critical elements of modern healthcare organisations provides an excellent marketing and promotional resource.

A second important, but related, consideration is simple survival. The NHS, like all public sector organisations, is subject to spending reviews, funding cuts and financial restraints. If seen as a 'nice to have' or optional extra, the knowledge and library service could easily be earmarked for funding reductions or more serious cost cutting measures. By demonstrating that the knowledge and library service is a business-critical function of the organisation, providing a net benefit in terms of bringing innovations and efficiencies through its core services, there is a far greater argument for looking elsewhere to find financial savings.

In 2014, Health Education England launched the Knowledge for Healthcare strategy, setting the direction for the development of NHS knowledge and library services in England. A key strand of the Quality Workstream was to revise and refresh an existing impact tool, which had been made available for NHS knowledge and library services as described by Weightman et al. (2009). Despite the availability of this earlier tool, the evidence showed that many library and knowledge services were not routinely measuring the impacts made by their service. NHS library and knowledge specialists often confused feedback relating to user satisfaction and impact (Ayre et al., 2018). Nevertheless, a systematic review confirmed that where health librarians collected evidence of their impact, they were able to demonstrate positive impacts across multiple outcomes (Brettle and Maden, 2016).

A task and finish group was set up to review and update the Value and Impact Toolkit with the aim of addressing some of the challenges identified above. The methodology used by the task and finish group included a literature search, a baseline survey on the use of the existing toolkit and development and piloting of a questionnaire (Ayre et al., 2018). The questionnaire was later validated (Urquhart and Brettle, 2022), confirming the reliability of the tool in measuring the impact of NHS knowledge and library services. The refreshed Value and Impact Toolkit (Health Education England, 2016b) includes the validated generic questionnaire, an interview schedule, a template for the creation of impact narratives and a resource presenting a range of material useful in measuring value and impact. The working group included a recommendation around the administration of the questionnaire, suggesting that better responses result from a focus on one specific incident (or use) rather than any more general use of the library (Ayre et al., 2018). The questionnaire focuses on impact as both immediate and probable future outcomes.

Since the launch of the Toolkit there has been a considerable increase in the generation of impact evidence across the NHS in England to demonstrate the value of knowledge and library services. A survey was carried out in Spring 2019 to determine how many services had implemented the Toolkit – with a response rate of 100%, this survey showed that 75% of knowledge and library services were using the Toolkit and of these, 80% were using the generic questionnaire. Slightly fewer services (64%) were gathering qualitative data through interviewing and the development of impact case studies. In general, the development of impact case studies has become the most powerful means of demonstrating the impact and value of knowledge and library services across England. NHS librarians are encouraged to submit case studies to a national repository, with over 300 accepted to date. Many of these narratives have been developed into impact vignettes.

Impact data only reaches its full potential value if it is used to evidence the critical functions that knowledge and library services fulfil in the NHS and healthcare environment. Gilroy and Turner (2018) demonstrated how knowledge and library services were championing their organisational impact at local level. Research showed that knowledge and library services were using impact evidence and data in a variety of ways, including in annual reports and promotional materials, to highlight their value to stakeholders. The use of quotes from stakeholders who have benefited from the use of knowledge and library services is an important part of the case study development. The vignettes invariably include the name and job role of the individual who has worked with the knowledge and library service and benefited from the resulting impacts. This recommendation is used in promotional material addressing peers at both national and local level, ensuring the role of health knowledge and library services is visible to high level decision makers influencing thinking and policy.

The Quality and Improvement Outcomes Framework for NHS Funded Library and Knowledge Services in England (Outcomes Framework), launched in 2019, brings further attention to the measurement and use of impact within NHS knowledge and library services. Self-evaluation against the Outcomes Framework is mandated for all NHS organisations holding an Education Contract with Health Education England and a 97% return rate was achieved for the baseline self-evaluation in 2021. This included 100% of those organisations with an internally hosted knowledge and library service, providing an excellent snapshot of NHS knowledge and library services in England during 2021. The Outcomes Framework consists of six outcomes, with the theme for Outcome 6 being 'Knowledge and library specialists demonstrate that their services make a positive impact on healthcare'. The indicators align well with the use of the Value and Impact Toolkit outlined above. Although use of the Toolkit itself is not obligatory, and progress against the Outcomes Framework can be achieved using other routes, the Toolkit provides a tried and tested means of collecting impact data and using it to promote the service. During the baseline self-evaluation, many services demonstrated the use of the Toolkit in the narrative and evidence they provided.

The baseline self-evaluation was validated by members of Health Education England's Knowledge and Library team to ensure it was consistent and provided a reliable baseline. Early results from the validation indicate that services were able to demonstrate a higher level of development against Outcome 6 (impact) than any of the other Outcomes.

The Outcomes Framework is intended to be a tool for continuous service improvement and it is recognised that NHS knowledge and library services have work still to do around demonstrating impact. Nevertheless, this strong starting position suggests that impact is already a key concern for many NHS knowledge and library specialists in England, with much work underway using the Value and Impact Toolkit and other mechanisms.

Making Alignment a Priority (MAP) Community: peer support for impact work

Making Alignment a Priority (MAP) is a community of practice established in 2008 to support knowledge and library services in demonstrating impact. The aim of the community was twofold: first, to help librarians to understand local, regional and national NHS priorities; and secondly, to enable librarians to showcase examples of library impact aligned with these priorities.

Aligning with strategic drivers

MAP emerged at a time when it was becoming clear in the NHS in England that knowledge and library services needed to align with the strategic objectives of their host organisation. The impact agenda was driven by a need to justify organisational investment in knowledge and library services – a need that continues today.

To be able to successfully influence and advocate the value of knowledge and library services, MAP recognised that speaking the same language as strategic decision makers was imperative. In order to do this, it was vital that librarians understood key strategic drivers ('drivers for change') that were of concern at senior and board level in their organisations. Together, MAP members produced summaries of key strategic drivers for a librarian audience. As an example, in 2015, The King's Fund published *Implementing the NHS Five Year Forward View: Aligning Policies with the Plan* (The King's Fund, 2015), a report that examined the implementation of the *NHS Five Year Forward View* (NHS England, 2014). Members of the MAP Community published a summary of the report. Highlighted within the summary were opportunities for demonstrating impact:

> The vision of the NHS becoming a learning organisation … is a great
> opportunity to expand and promote our skill sets and services.
> (MAP Community, 2015)

Summarising the report and reframing the findings in the context of knowledge and library services enabled NHS librarians to consider what implications the report might have for them and how they might use it to leverage impact activities to be more meaningful to strategic decision makers in their organisation.

Peer-to-peer support

The MAP Community continued to evolve over the following years. As Health Education England's Knowledge for Healthcare framework was implemented (Health Education England, 2014; Health Education England, 2021a) and #AMillionDecisions (Day and Goswami, 2020), a joint campaign led by CILIP Health Libraries Group and Health Education England, launched, MAP developed to work alongside these national programmes that had similar aims.

An appetite grew within the MAP Community to learn from each other about impact. What impact activities were other services involved in? What had they learned along the way? Examples of practice were shared. A series of workshops was facilitated across England by MAP members to share peer-to-peer learning around impact work in NHS libraries. Common challenges, such as dealing with shifting strategic priorities and service pressures, were discussed. Attendees were encouraged to develop their own local impact planning during the workshop, with accompanying materials, practical exercises and peer support. One workshop attendee commented on how the workshop had informed their local strategic approach:

> We are currently working on developing a new impact strategy at my trust. I have been able to apply what I learnt from the training to this task.
>
> (Workshop feedback, 2019)

Another workshop attendee commented on how the learning from MAP had influenced them to develop processes to capture impact:

> We are now looking at sending follow-up emails to users a month after they've attended training or receive a literature search. Whilst we have always collected initial feedback, we had never checked how the service has impacted practice.
>
> (Workshop feedback, 2019)

MAP workshops supported attendees to develop practical approaches to demonstrating impact and enabled librarians to assemble in pursuit of a common aim.

An evolving community of practice

The evolution of MAP as a community of practice illustrates the importance of member-led networks in librarianship. MAP was conceived in response to sector-wide discussions and concerns about impact. Its members worked in knowledge and library services in different organisations, however, collectively they supported each other in pursuit of a common aim. MAP members developed materials and tools to support members in the endeavour to demonstrate impact and became a vehicle for peer support. Although the global COVID-19 pandemic forced members to concentrate on other priorities, the challenge of demonstrating impact remains. MAP and other communities of practice remain vital to librarians to enable skills development, problem solving and collective knowledge-sharing to address common challenges.

Conclusion

NHS knowledge and library specialists use impact data in a variety of different ways. Some examples were noted by Gilroy and Turner (2018), including the use of impact quotes in social media promotional campaigns, annual reports and other service documentation to inform discussions with senior staff and healthcare teams and for other promotional activity.

At a national level, impact data is vital for senior leaders to promote the need for the skills of knowledge and library specialists in organisational decision-making, particularly to those parts of the NHS that currently do not benefit from access to these highly specialist services.

The NHS invests £50m a year in NHS library and knowledge services in England. Data is great but a story is powerful beyond any graph or table. It is absolutely vital to have impact stories to hand, in our back pocket, ready to tell.

(Sue Lacey Bryant, Chief Knowledge Officer and National Lead for NHS Knowledge and Library Services)

Stories about the impact of health libraries are often presented graphically in the form of vignettes. These provide excellent snapshots of the individual impacts of knowledge and library services in a specific situation, but Health Education England was interested in developing a larger scale narrative to illustrate the high level impacts of knowledge and library services across the country. To address this challenge, Health Education England commissioned a health economist to work with the knowledge and library teams to develop a value proposition for NHS knowledge and library services. The intention was to progress from the many individual stories of the impact of knowledge and library services to establish a larger scale perspective. Whereas the tools contained within the Value and Impact Toolkit take a critical incident approach, focusing in on a specific instance of a service offer in one defined situation, the value proposition is intended to offer a broader statement about the impact, specifically the economic benefit, of NHS knowledge and library services across England.

Economics by Design, the company commissioned to work with Health Education England, worked through a number of impact case studies in developing the proposition and led a workshop with impact case study authors to explore the services offered by NHS knowledge and library specialists in more detail. A literature search was also undertaken to identify the impacts, particularly around financial and time saving benefits, of healthcare library services. This highlighted consistent evidence nationally and internationally for a clear economic benefit associated with the use of healthcare library services, with a study from the Wirral (Hartfiel et al., 2020) confirming the pattern for NHS knowledge and library services in England.

The study also included cross mapping of impact case studies with services from organisations performing well in the Care Quality Commission (CQC) inspections. Data from interviews with knowledge and library service managers was combined with information from Health Education England's annual statistics returns from NHS knowledge and library services to inform the study.

The resulting report, *NHS Funded Library and Knowledge Services in England – Value Proposition: The Gift of Time* (Economics by Design, 2020), provides an overview of the economic benefits offered by NHS knowledge and library services to the NHS in England, together with recommendations for NHS organisations to maximise these benefits. The report confirms some of the key themes highlighted by the impact case studies collected at local level by services. Namely that NHS knowledge and library specialists save the time of healthcare professionals. The report uses the image of the 'gift of time' to describe how the work undertaken by healthcare knowledge and library specialists releases more time for healthcare professionals to spend on patient care and other priorities.

In terms of economic benefits, the report makes use of statistical data and other research to estimate that, based on these time savings alone, NHS knowledge and library specialists may already be providing a net economic benefit of £77 million per annum to the NHS in England. This is after the costs of NHS staff and services have been accounted for.

The report was welcomed by Health Education England and CILIP and was presented to an All-Party Parliamentary Group for Libraries, resulting in an endorsement from a member of the group:

> Healthcare librarians and knowledge specialists do a wonderful job in collating important information and bridging research and frontline care. This valuable asset helps to facilitate knowledge-sharing within the NHS and provide better healthcare outcomes.
>
> (Gill Furniss, Member of Parliament for Sheffield Brightside and Hillsborough)

This example shows how impact data and associated information collected at a local level can be used to demonstrate the importance of knowledge and library services nationally.

The use of metrics, and both quantitative and qualitative data, to evidence the value and impact of services is an invaluable tool for knowledge and library professionals.

Within the field of healthcare, these tools have been used to great effect at both local and national level to demonstrate the business-critical nature of the services provided by knowledge and library specialists to the wider healthcare system.

References

Ayre, S., Brettle, A., Gilroy, D., Knock, D., Mitchelmore, R., Pattison, S., Smith, S. and Turner, J. (2018) Developing a Generic Tool to Routinely Measure the Impact of Health Libraries, *Health Information and Libraries Journal*, **35** (3), 227–45.

Brettle, A. and Maden, M. (2016) *What Evidence is there to Support the*

Employment of Professionally Trained Library, Information and Knowledge Workers? A systematic Scoping Review of the Evidence.
www.researchgate.net/publication/301626933_What_evidence_is_there_
to_support_the_employment_of_trained_and_professionally_registered_
library_information_and_knowledge_workers_A_systematic_scoping_
review_of_the_evidence.

Day, A. and Goswami, L. (2020) Driving Change with Evidence and Knowledge: Transforming Knowledge Services for the NHS Across England, *Business Information Review*, **37** (1), 10–18.

Earl. S., Carden. F. and Smutylo, T. (2001) *Outcome Mapping: Building Learning and Reflection into Development Programs*, International Development Research Centre.

Economics by Design (2020) *NHS Funded Library and Knowledge Services in England – Value Proposition: The Gift of Time.* www.hee.nhs.uk/our-work/library-knowledge-services/value-proposition-gift-time.

Fricker, A. (2017) *Building Better Metrics – Drive Better Conversations.* Paper presented at the International Congress of Medical Librarianship (ICML) and European Association for Health Information and Libraries (EAHIL) 2017 Conference, Dublin, June 12–16.

Gann, L. B. and Pratt, G. F. (2013) Using Library Search Service Metrics to Demonstrate Library Value and Manage Workload, *Journal of the Medical Library Association*, **101** (3), 227–9.

Gilroy. D. and Turner. J. (2018) *Showcasing the Impact of Health Libraries in England.* Paper presented at the European Association for Health Information and libraries (EAHIL) Conference, Cardiff, July 9–13. https://eahilcardiff2018.wordpress.com/programme-2.

Hartfiel, N., Sadera, G., Treadway, V., Lawrence, C. and Tudor Edwards, R. (2020) A Clinical Librarian in a Hospital Critical Care Unit May Generate a Positive Return on Investment, *Health Information and Libraries Journal*, **38** (2), 97–112.

Health Education England (2014) *Knowledge for Healthcare: A Development Framework.*
www.hee.nhs.uk/sites/default/files/documents/Knowledge_for_healthcare_
a_development_framework_2014.pdf.

Health Education England (2016a) *Principles for Metrics Report and Recommendations.* https://library.hee.nhs.uk/binaries/content/assets/lks/
quality-and-impact/value-and-impact-toolkit/value-and-impact-
toolkit/metrics-principles-report-final-2016.pdf.

Health Education England, (2016b) *Value and Impact Toolkit.*
https://library.hee.nhs.uk/quality-and-impact/value-and-impact/value-and-
impact-toolkit.

Health Education England (2017) *Statistics Toolkit.*
https://library.hee.nhs.uk/quality-and-impact/data-and-statistics/statistics-toolbox.

Health Education England (2019) *Quality and Improvement Outcomes Framework for NHS Funded Library and Knowledge Services in England.*
https://library.hee.nhs.uk/binaries/content/assets/lks/quality-and-impact/quality-and-improvement-outcomes-framework-documentation/quality-and-improvement-framework-2019.pdf.

Health Education England (2020) NHS Library and Knowledge Services in England: Recommendations to Improve the Staff Ratio for the Number of Qualified Library and Knowledge Specialists Per Member of the NHS Workforce.
www.hee.nhs.uk/sites/default/files/documents/HEE%20LKS%20Staff%20Ratio%20Policy%20January%202020.pdf.

Health Education England (2021a) *Knowledge for Healthcare: Mobilising Evidence; Sharing Knowledge; Improving Outcomes. A Strategic Framework for NHS Knowledge and Library Services 2021–2026.*
www.hee.nhs.uk/our-work/knowledge-for-healthcare.

Health Education England (2021b) *NHS Funded Knowledge and Library Services in England: Highlights 2020–21: Staffing.*
https://library.hee.nhs.uk/binaries/content/assets/lks/quality-and-impact/annual-statistical-return/staffing-2020-21-infographic.pdf.

Health Education England (2021c) *Evaluation Framework.*
https://library.hee.nhs.uk/quality-and-impact/evaluation-framework.

International Organization for Standardization (2014) BS ISO 16439:2014. *Methods and Procedures for Assessing the Impact of Libraries.* BSI.

Killick, S. (2021) *The Evolution and Impact of Library Data.* In 14th International Conference on Performance Measurement in Libraries, 2–4 Nov. http://oro.open.ac.uk/80030.

Loughborough University (2001) *Library and Information Statistical Tables for the United Kingdom: Statistics from the NHS Regional Librarians Group,* Loughborough University.

MAP Community (2015) *Implementing the NHS Five Year Forward View: Aligning Policies with the Plan.*
www.lihnnhs.info/maptoolkit/2015/12/03/1147.

Muller, J. (2019) *The Tyranny of Metrics,* Princeton University Press.

NHS England, (2014) *NHS Five Year Forward View.* www.england.nhs.uk/wp-content/uploads/2014/10/5yfv-web.pdf.

Oxford University Press (2022) *Definition of 'Metric',* OED Online.
www.oed.com/view/Entry/117657.

Showers, B. (2015) Metrics: Counting What Really Matters, *CILIP Update*, February, 42–4.

Streatfield, D. (2012) Impact Planning and Assessment of Public Libraries: A Country Level Perspective, *Performance Measurement and Metrics*, **13** (1), 8–14.

The King's Fund (2015) Implementing the NHS Five Year Forward View: Aligning Policies with the Plan. www.kingsfund.org.uk/publications/implementing-nhs-five-year-forward-view.

Urquhart, C. and Brettle, A. (2022) Validation of a Generic Impact Survey for Use by Health Library Services Indicates the Reliability of the Questionnaire, *Health Information and Library Journal*, **39** (4), 323–35.

Weightman, A., Urquhart, C., Spink, S. and Thomas, R. (2009) The Value and Impact of Information Provided Through Library Services for Patient Care: Developing Guidance for Best Practice, *Health Information and Library Journal*, **26** (1), 63–71.

Workshop Feedback (2019) Unpublished feedback collected from MAP Workshop Facilitators.

11

Reflective Practice in Healthcare Settings

Tracey Pratchett, Siobhan Linsey and Rachel Cooke

Introduction

The ability to reflect on what we do and how we do it is an essential strategy for health professionals working in healthcare organisations. The art of reflection enables practitioners to improve patient care, develop skills and knowledge, improve the quality of services and enhance organisational development. Many higher education courses for healthcare professionals include reflective practice as part of the curriculum. The ability to reflect continues to be relevant throughout careers as it is embedded within ongoing professional development, including revalidation, team debriefs and personal reflection on experiences.

The purpose of this chapter is to help knowledge and library staff to develop these skills. It will encourage the reader to consider the importance of being a reflective practitioner for personal development and to understand how to provide services that also enable healthcare professionals to develop their skills. Furthermore, we will explore how a reflective practice approach is used for team reflection in both healthcare teams and knowledge and library services to facilitate ongoing improvement.

As this book aims to be a practical guide, there will be a summary of some key theories relating to the discipline and models that can be applied to improve reflective practice, alongside some hints and exercises for writing reflectively. A number of case studies are included from people working in knowledge and library services to provide real-life examples of how reflective practice is integral to healthcare professionals working in healthcare organisations.

Theories of reflective practice

There is a huge body of literature relating to reflective practice. This chapter will not provide an exhaustive list but will focus on a couple of theories that will be useful for putting reflective practice into perspective.

The Chartered Institute for Professional Development

The Chartered Institute for Professional Development (CIPD) defines reflective practice as 'the foundation of professional development' (CIPD, 2018). It highlights that adopting an approach of reflective practice helps professionals to make meaning from experiences and develop practical strategies for personal growth and organisational impact. Reflective practice is a personal learning journey, enabling practitioners to consider what they can learn from their experiences and develop plans to make changes in the future.

Donald Schon

In his book *The Reflective Practitioner*, Schon (1991) states that reflection can happen in two ways. First, he describes 'reflection-in-action', which is a process of reflecting during an experience or activity. This may happen unconsciously and is likely to be an immediate response to the situation; by reflecting in the moment it is possible to make changes to practice as a direct result of reflecting on experience. An example of this would be when a knowledge and library staff member is delivering a teaching session to a group of nurses, but the projector in the room stops working. To deal with the issue, the trainer deviates from the original plan and adapts the session by introducing a different approach to delivering the content. This type of reflection is instinctive rather than structured; immediate reflection on experience is used to make changes in the moment. It is an adaptive and organic approach to reflection.

Schon (1991) goes on to describe 'reflection-on-action', which happens after an experience has taken place. This form of reflection is a conscious and in-depth process that involves consulting with others and reviewing evidence before making changes to practice. An example of this is where a knowledge and library staff member delivers a new training programme over four months that includes four sessions. During the programme, a structured reflective activity takes places after each session and trainees are surveyed to evaluate their experience. At the end of the programme the evaluation forms are reviewed and the reflective notes are considered. This combination of data is then used to make recommendations that will improve the training programme. This is a more structured approach to reflective practice.

David Kolb

David Kolb (1984) talks about experiential learning as being a cyclical process. After the experience, you reflect on it, then move into the abstract conceptualisation stage where you form new ideas and theories based on your reflections. The final stage of this process involves applying the new ideas to practice with active experimentation (Figure 11.1).

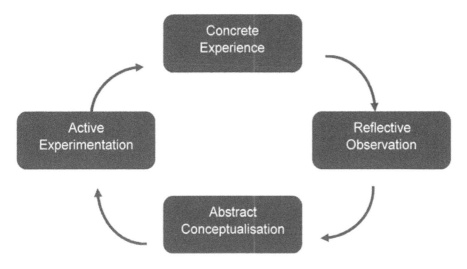

Figure 11.1 *Adapted from David Kolb's* Experiential Learning (1984), 48

This active experimentation informs a new concrete experience. Using the example of delivering a training programme, the second year of delivering the programme becomes a new concrete experience incorporating the improvements. The modified programme now goes through the same cycle of reflection, ideas generation and active experimentation to identify any further changes or refinements. Kolb defines this as an ongoing cycle of learning from experience, with reflection and observing what has happened as a basis for generating new ideas and applying learning to practice.

Reflective practice for knowledge and library professionals

Reflective practice is as relevant for knowledge and library professionals as it is for other healthcare professionals. Professional bodies, such as CILIP in the UK, encourage members to reflect as they work towards achieving professional registration. Candidates are asked to reflect on their personal performance, the organisational context of their service and the wider professional context of library services (CILIP, 2020). Continual reflection ensures that knowledge and library staff continue to develop and improve their personal knowledge and skills.

Approaches to reflective practice

Reflective practice can be applied in many different ways. There is no single way of applying the theories to our personal practice and we will all develop our own personal preference as to how we reflect. In the knowledge and library services profession, it is important that we develop an approach to reflection that suits our own way of working. Miller, Ford and Yang (2020) identify a number of approaches to reflective practice. Practitioners may choose a single approach or use a combination of these (Table 11.1).

Table 11.1 *Approaches to reflective writing* (adapted from Miller, Ford and Yang, 2020)

Approach	Description
Reflection without recording	Pros – Useful when time is short. Cons – Relies on memory to follow through.
Reflecting alone and capturing the learning	Pros – Outputs are recorded for future use. Cons – More time-consuming.
Talking through with another person	Pros – Use a mentor, coach or colleagues to talk things through and generate new insights. Cons – Need to consider confidentiality.
Talking through with a group of people	Pros – Shared reflection via peer support groups, such as action learning sets, can enable rich discussion. Cons – Need to consider confidentiality.
Initially reflecting alone followed by talking with others	Pros – Initial individualised reflection followed by reflecting with others can deepen insights. Cons – Need to consider confidentiality.

Models to aid reflective writing

Reflective writing is the process of formally capturing learning and identifying areas of improvement. CILIP embeds the process of reflection into its routes to professional registration and provides guidance on reflective writing for candidates. CILIP defines reflective writing as an opportunity to outline:

> Reflective writing is a technique to capture experiences, opinions, events or new information. It is a process to help you to explore your learning and gain self-knowledge. Most importantly it is your personal reaction to the situations you encounter and is invaluable when aiming to get the most out of your learning experiences.
>
> (CILIP, 2020)

There are many models that can be used and adapted to aid reflective writing. This chapter will consider three models that you can use for capturing learning from reflection. All models include a number of questions under headings that can be used to deliver deeper insights.

The STAR framework

CILIP (2020) recommends that candidates may wish to use the STAR framework (Table 11.2) to structure their pieces of reflective writing. This framework was originally developed to support candidates in answering structured interview questions (Mindtools, 2022). The questions prompt the reflector to explore the situation from different perspectives to extract learning.

Table 11.2 *The STAR framework,* reproduced from CILIP (2020)

Situation Questions	Task Questions	Action Questions	Result Questions
What was involved? Who was involved? What was the challenge? What was the issue?	What was the objective? What was the goal?	What did you do? Why did you do it that way? What are your thoughts about the action that you took? What are your feelings about the action that you took?	What changed? What was the outcome? What did you learn?

Terry Borton

Terry Borton (1970) developed a simple model for reflective practice that includes three simple questions (Table 11.3). By working through each of these questions, a reflective practitioner can think deeply and critically about an incident or activity and identify areas for improvement that can be applied to practice.

Table 11.3 *Borton's reflective practice model*

What happened?	What was the task? Who was involved? Who asked you to do it?
So what?	Why is it important? Who was impacted? What are the outcomes?
What next?	What worked/didn't work so well? What will you change? How will you apply the learning?

Graham Gibbs
The Gibbs model (1988) includes six stages to guide reflection (Table 11.4). It builds on the Borton model and splits the analysis section 'so what' into more specific areas. The reflective practitioner is guided to consider feelings and this model is particularly suited to healthcare professions who need to consider the impact of incidents on themselves, their patients and their colleagues.

Table 11.4 *Gibbs' reflective practice model*

Step 1 – Description	Step 2 – Feelings	Step 3 – Evaluation
Set the scene and provide some context.	How did you feel before and after the event? How did others feel?	Objectively consider what went well and what did not go so well.
Step 4 – Analysis	**Step 5 – Conclusions**	**Step 6 – Action Plan**
Analysis attempts to explain why the experience was positive or negative and should be the longest part of your reflection.	What have you learned and how will you apply this to future experiences?	What specific actions can you take to build your knowledge and skills?

Tips for reflecting

These models provide guidance questions to enable deeper learning and can be adapted to suit your personal needs and preferences. If the structured approach starts to hinder your writing rather than enabling it, either try a different model, create your own useful questions to guide reflection or try free writing. Each model includes prompt questions that are there to encourage deeper critical thinking and to help you analyse a situation from different angles. When using these models, it is important to ensure that your writing includes a minimal amount of description, with the main focus being on the analysis of the situation, identifying improvements or focusing on what went well to incorporate into future practice.

Everyone has a different approach to reflective writing, there is no prescriptive approach. It is important that you develop your own approach to reflective practice for it to be successful. The main thing is to focus on the meaning behind the experience and to identify learning that can be applied to future practice. Whilst written reflection is often the most accepted approach and is usually the preferred method for formal education, it is important that practitioners find an approach that suits them to ensure that reflective practice becomes an ongoing habit.

Try the models listed above, but if you find that they are getting in the way of your writing flow, maybe try a different model or create your own by selecting the questions that are meaningful for you. If the models don't work for you, set a short time limit of 10 minutes and try writing without any structure. Exploring the incident that you want to reflect on by free writing can help you to move beyond writer's block.

If you want to get the most out of adopting a reflective approach to improve your practice, try to dedicate specific time to reflect. By dedicating regular time for reflection at the end of the day, or each week, you can start to build a habit where reflection becomes a natural part of your way of working. Some people find that journaling can be a good way of developing a habit. If you want to reflect on a specific incident, try to capture your thoughts when it is fresh in your mind – you can revisit at a later date to evaluate and analyse what happened.

Not everyone finds writing is the best way to reflect. If you are struggling with writing, why not try video or audio recordings to capture your reflections? When you are developing a reflective practice for yourself, it does not matter what approach you adopt, it just needs to work for you. Of course, if you are reflecting as part of a formal process for education or professional registration, you may need to develop your reflective writing skills.

Whatever approach you adopt, just remember that your reflections should not be wholly descriptive but should analyse what happened with a view to developing actions that can be applied to future practice. When reflecting for education or professional registration, ensure that you focus on the meaning behind the reflection. Think about the difference that you made and consider your personal impact. Finally, consider what changes will you take forward for future practice.

Activity

Now it is time for you to have a go at reflective writing. Choose an experience that you would like to reflect on. This could be something that happened on your course, such as a presentation you have delivered, or something that happened at work, such as a project you are working on.

- Select one of the three models and spend 10 minutes writing about the experience using the prompts provided. Write quickly, working through as many questions as you can.
- Once the 10 minutes are over, consider how useful the model was.
- Were there any challenges?
- Could you adapt the model by adding or removing questions to make it work for you?

Now test a different model to reflect on another experience and assess how that one works for you.

Reflective practice for knowledge and library teams

As well as using reflective practice as part of your own personal development, you may find that the work team you join also uses reflection to inform and develop the services it provides. In healthcare, it is important that teams reflect together and this is often done in an informal way. However, there are two ways that healthcare teams (including knowledge and library services) should use more systematic approaches to reflection:

1 When something doesn't go as expected or there is an adverse event.
2 When working to improve or develop a process or service, for example, quality improvement.

It is by reflecting together in a focused way that teams can learn and improve what they are seeking to do.

Tools for team reflective learning

When something doesn't go as expected, there is a need to find out why this happened and to learn lessons in order to try and avoid the same thing happening again (Milton, 2010, 2). This should be done in an organised way and there are a number of tools and processes that can be used.

After action reviews

One tool that is straightforward to use is the after action review (AAR) process. AARs originated in the US armed forces, where they were used to gain understanding and reflection after an incident. AARs are now used in many industries worldwide including the NHS (Collison and Parcell, 2001,132).

AARs are a facilitated process that a group of people or a team involved in an event or incident can use to reflect together on what actually happened. The process involves just four questions that the group will answer together:

1 What was expected to happen?
2 What actually happened?
3 Why was there a difference?
4 What can we learn from this?

AARs are also one of the tools in the knowledge mobiliser's toolkit to support programmes and projects, building reflection and moments of pause part way or at the end of a project. AARs are also used by NHS knowledge and library specialists in this context (Health Education England, 2021). For further information about AARs and knowledge mobilisation see Chapter 5.

Reflection for service improvement

Teams also reflect when developing new ways of working, improving or changing an existing service or process. In healthcare, this is known as quality improvement (Care Quality Commission, 2018). You will find that most NHS organisations are involved in quality improvement and will often have a team that leads or supports others in the organisation to carry this out. In the same way as it is important to reflect when something doesn't go according to plan, reflection should also be part of the quality improvement process, as the team involved reflects on the changes it has made and considers what it should do next.

> Improvers are reflective practitioners, comfortable using a range of evaluative methods to better understand whether changes are improvements or not. Reflectors are able to learn from experiences both in the moment and systematically over time taking multiple perspectives on their own actions.
>
> (Lucas and Nacer, 2015, 13)

Plan, do, study, act

Healthcare knowledge and library teams also need to improve, adapt and modify the services they provide and can use the same tools as other healthcare teams to help them reflect as they develop their services. One improvement tool that is common to a number of quality improvement methodologies and has reflective practice embedded in it is the 'plan, do, study, act' (PDSA) cycle (NHS England 2022).

As the name implies, with this method you identify what change or improvement you want to test and how you will identify if the improvement is effective. You carry out the improvement and you then look at what you have done to see if it was effective, reflecting on what further changes you may need to make or whether the improvement is ready to be implemented. One improvement may involve a number of PDSA cycles.

Case Study 11.1 below is an example of how the library and knowledge service at Surrey and Sussex Healthcare NHS Trust carried out an AAR to reflect and learn together after something didn't go as they expected. Having identified changes they thought they needed to make, they carried out PDSA cycles to reflect, learn and continue to make further changes.

Case Study 11.1: Using AARs and PDSA cycles to improve the LKS involvement in junior doctor induction

Team/project lead: Library and Knowledge Service (LKS) / Rachel Cooke
Trust: Surrey and Sussex Healthcare NHS Trust
Target group: Junior doctors

In 2018, the hospital changed the way that the large summer inductions of new doctors in postgraduate training were run. The LKS team felt that their participation in the induction could have gone better so carried out an AAR.

The AAR helped them understand why things did not go as well as they had expected. Most importantly, by reflecting on this together they were able to identify ways that they could try and improve their approach to the junior doctor induction the following year.

The AAR was documented and in 2019 the team revisited the AAR and put in place some of the changes that had been identified. The team decided to continue the process of reflection and learning using PDSA cycles to help them take a systematic approach to their reflection and to continue to make modifications. This was possible as there were two cohorts of new doctors starting – the induction of the smaller group of about 30 doctors took place first, followed by the larger group of over 100 doctors the following week. The team used this as an opportunity to carry out two PDSA cycles, one per induction event.

Key themes: improving services, using improvement approaches

Reflective practice for the healthcare professions

Reflective practice is essential for healthcare professionals to ensure that they improve patient care, maintain safety, develop their skills, demonstrate competence, look after their personal wellbeing and continue to learn from mistakes and good practice. As a knowledge and library professional working in a healthcare setting, you may be required to provide services that facilitate reflective practice for a range of healthcare professionals at different stages of their careers.

Expectations of professional bodies in healthcare

In the same way that CILIP embeds reflective practice in the journey to professional registration for its members, healthcare professionals are expected to reflect throughout their careers. The Academy of Medical Royal Colleges and the Conference of Postgraduate Medical Deans (COPMeD) (2018) define reflective practice as the 'process whereby an individual thinks analytically about anything relating to their professional practice with the intention of gaining insight and using the lessons learned to maintain good practice or make improvements where possible.'

The Nursing and Midwifery Council (2018) Code of Conduct has embedded the importance of reflection within revalidation, where nursing colleagues are expected to evidence their ability to practice safely and effectively. The General Medical Council (GMC, 2018) provides detailed guidelines to support reflective practice throughout the career pathway, from medical student to consultant roles. Through revalidation, doctors reflect, demonstrating their fitness to practice and identify ways that practice can be improved or developed. The Health and Care Professions Council (2021) highlights the importance of reflective practice for professions, not only to develop insights and learning with regard to practicing healthcare, but also developing bonds within teams.

Reflective practice for healthcare teams

As well as reflecting as part of their individual practice, healthcare teams often practice reflection as a team to improve the delivery of healthcare and to investigate when things go wrong. There are lots of professionals involved in the care of an individual patient and team meetings, case review panels and Schwartz Rounds are all methods that can help teams to work together to improve patient care. Team debriefing and clinical supervision (Bifarin and Stonehouse, 2017) provide support that can aid reflection and provide a confidential space to discuss work, to improve practice and patient care. Debriefing in the clinical environment enables a whole team perspective, which supports both personal and professional needs (Clark and McLean, 2019). Schwartz Rounds (Point of Care Foundation, 2022) are also a way in which people can reflect on the emotional aspects of working in healthcare. Based around a topic, three stories are shared and the discussion is opened up to all present to share their experiences in a safe, facilitated space. Knowledge and library staff often support these sessions by providing reading lists linked to the topic, promoting the events and acting as a facilitator or steering group member.

Knowledge and library services supporting reflective practice

There are many ways in which knowledge and library professionals can facilitate reflective practice for healthcare staff. Knowledge and library services provide reading lists, books, access to electronic resources that have embedded elements for reflective practice, deliver training sessions and provide feedback on pieces of reflective writing. Case Study 11.2 below outlines how a knowledge and library professional developed a reflective practice training session for their healthcare staff.

Case Study 11.2: Creating a reflective practice session in a healthcare library

Team/project lead: Trust Library Services / Bethan Morgan

Trust: Manchester University NHS Foundation Trust
Target group: Physiotherapists, nurses and senior clinicians
I decided to design a training session on reflective practice as I felt that this was a significant gap in the information skills training offered to healthcare staff by the library services. Initially, I spoke with colleagues in nursing education about whether this would be of interest and to see what kind of content would be most useful. I also asked colleagues from other healthcare libraries about their experiences of running sessions on reflective practice. I immediately received great advice, as well as numerous offers to shadow sessions. This helped to inform the structure and content of my session.

Reflective practice is valuable for all healthcare staff, so my session is aimed at a multi-professional audience. Indeed, attendees so far have included physiotherapists, nurses and senior clinicians. However, in the future, I would like to tailor the content to specific audiences, such as nurses undertaking revalidation, to ensure that attendees find it as useful as possible.

My aim for the session is for it to be interactive and engaging. However, reflection can be very personal and I did not want attendees to feel uncomfortable or forced into sharing their own reflections. As a result, I share my own reflection on an imagined scenario using the Gibbs model. Attendees are then prompted to discuss its strengths and weaknesses. Following on from this, they are given time to write their own reflections. The discussion afterwards is focused on how they found the process of writing. The feedback for this activity has been positive and attendees are able to use what they have written in their CPD portfolios if they wish.

Overall, the response has been encouraging, suggesting there is a remit for healthcare libraries to provide training on reflective practice.
Key themes: training, tailored content, reflective writing practice

Creative writing and reflective practice

Frameworks that personalise reflective practice can be most effective for allowing experiences and challenging encounters to be processed and turned into knowledge.

Reflective writing is not only about gathering the facts of a situation, but also how a member of staff understands their performance:

> Reflective notes do not need to capture full factual details of an experience. They should focus on the learning or actions taken from a case or situation. Reflection is personal and there is no one way to reflect.

(GMC, 2018)

Knowledge and library services staff can bolster this by facilitating reflective writing sessions that enable staff to process incidents in a way that not only supports formal learning (providing evidence to support revalidation/professional portfolios, etc.), but also addresses the emotional impact sometimes left by incidents at work, which can affect staff wellbeing and morale. These sessions are an investment in staff, helping to prevent burnout, and maintain retention for positive organisational impact.

Creative and critical analysis of an event

A blend of creative and critical analysis can help to achieve holistic reflective awareness. Creative writing techniques can be applied to allow staff to work through emotions and critical analysis can then affirm what went well, what can be improved and territories of new knowledge. Both are skills and behaviours for self-awareness.

Poetry in health libraries

There is a growing drive for healthcare knowledge and library services to use poetry to encourage reflection in staff, either through making poetry accessible to read in digital or hardcopy versions or through the provision of writing workshops, creating a space for mindful, expressive writing to support self-care.

The former is a natural extension of service provision, but the latter is more challenging: how many library professionals feel confident to facilitate such sessions? How can you justify the use of skilled time in this way to senior managers, illustrate impact or engage and exhibit benefits to staff?

Dr Eleanor Holmes and Sue Spencer

The 'Reflections on Clinical Encounters in Healthcare' workshop designed by Dr Eleanor Holmes and Sue Spencer is a good example of using both a guided writing framework activity and close reading of poetry and prose to support reflection for wellbeing. The session was developed when Dr Eleanor Holmes (NHS GP) was a GP tutor at Newcastle University Medical School delivering undergraduate teaching on Patient Centred Medicine and Sue Spencer (former district nurse and nurse educator at Northumbria University) was a Teaching Fellow in combined Honours at Newcastle University. Both are published poets (Dr Eleanor Holmes under the pen name Eliot North) as well as creative writing workshop facilitators, with Sue Spencer also Associate Editor for *BMJ Medical Humanities*.

The framework has been used by not only undergraduate medical students, but also healthcare professionals of all grades, as well as clinical teachers and academics at Newcastle University, University Hospital Bristol and Taunton and Somerset NHS Foundation Trust.

Central to the workshop is the use of a guided writing framework (Framework A – see Figure 11.2), which is read aloud by a facilitator. Attendees write in response to the prompts, revisiting a challenging incident and exploring it from different perspectives.

Framework A

The purpose of this framework is to enable you to explore an experience from clinical practice (or any experience that presents a challenge) within a creative writing exercise rather than simply report back on the facts. Creative writing allows you to engage your imagination, use imagery and metaphor, as well as pay close attention to the little details that can provide up-close observation.

Reflecting on the Clinical Encounter: A Guided Writing Framework
You are encouraged to name things; use Proper Nouns. Specific and concrete detail is good. Change the names of people and places to maintain anonymity.

(1) Scene Setting – Visual Imagination and Contextualisation
Close your eyes.
Recall a clinical encounter you have had/something that is bothering you at home or work. Take a minute to remember; we are going to paint a picture with words, using all your senses.
Open your eyes.
Where are you? What is the first thing you notice about this place?
How is the scene lit? What time of day is it? A line or two.
Who is in this place with you? If there is a group of people, how are they related?
What are they wearing? Do they have anything in their hands or nearby? What posture are they in? Elaborate for a line or two.
Is there a colour you associate with this scene? What does it make you think of?
Can you hear any snatches of music or background noise? (e.g., monitor beeps, tea trolley, traffic, radio) What does this sound like?

(2) Narrative Development – Characters and Backstory
What is happening in this scene? Why is it happening? Do all the players in the scene have the same 'why'? Elaborate for a few lines.
A camera lens clicks shut – it has captured an expression or gesture of your main subject. Describe the expression/gesture. How does this make you feel?
What words are being spoken? Give your main subject(s) a line of dialogue.
There is a detail you've not noticed until now (smell, texture, movement, etc.) – describe it here.
Bring someone you know (friend, family member, colleague) into the scene.
Who is this and how do they react? Elaborate for a line or two.

(3) Personal Development – Perspective Taking and Rehearsal
Imagine you are the main subject of this encounter. How do you feel? If you could change one thing about this encounter what would it be? What difference would it make? Expand for two or three lines.
Look over your writing. Finish with a couple of lines about what happens next for you after this scene or is happening just out of frame or in the wings.
If any words or phrases jump out at you, underline them and/or repeat them if you want to.

Figure 11.2 *Framework A: guided writing framework*

Facilitators would now encourage participants to read their work aloud (but if they do not wish to read their work this is OK) within a supportive atmosphere, giving feedback on insights gained through the exercise as well as any particular words or phrases that 'stand out' or could be explored further.

This exercise focuses on clinical narratives but there is no need to specify whether participants write prose, poetry or script – sometimes it is surprising what comes out when pen connects with paper!

Ideally, time would be given for people to read over and respond to their writing – with some examples of poetry and prose given to show what writing already exists exploring health themes or use these as jumping off points.

Authors
Framework devised and first utilised as a guided writing exercise within creative writing workshops on reflective practice for health professionals and students facilitated by Sue Spencer and Dr Eleanor Holmes, 2016, Newcastle-upon-Tyne, UK.

Acknowledgements
Writing Poems by Peter Sansom, Bloodaxe, 1993.
www.bloodaxebooks.com/ecs/product/writing-poems-405
The Poetry Toolkit – The Poetry Trust, 2010, available as a PDF download below.
https://bostonpoetry.files.wordpress.com/2013/09/toolkit-for-teachers.pdf

Special acknowledgement to the authors of the guided writing framework for their permission to use.

Figure 11.2 *Continued*

Case Study 11.3: Using a creative writing framework for reflective writing

Team/project lead: Library and Knowledge Service / Siobhan Linsey
Trust: Somerset NHS Foundation Trust
Target group: Admin and clinical teams
Inspired by this workshop [see Figure 11.2], the Outreach Librarian and Clinical Librarian at Somerset NHS Foundation Trust expanded its potential within the training offer of the library service. Having gained permission to use the framework established by Holmes and Spencer, the librarians revamped their Reflective Practice sessions, renaming the training 'Reflection for Professional Development – Not Just a Tick Box Exercise'.

The format followed three steps:

1 Creation of a psychologically safe space using an ice breaker activity and drawing up a 'group contract'.
2 Utilisation of the creative writing framework to address long-lasting emotional impact that clinical encounters can leave. Writing in response to the words of the framework being read aloud by the session lead, staff

revisited a challenging event personal to them, using techniques to engage the senses. Participants were encouraged to bring in a family member or colleague (often an authority figure), which allows them to appraise the situation. They were prompted to put themselves in the place of the main subject of the situation (e.g., the patient) and to view the situation from their perspective. This served to facilitate the processing of events in order to step back and objectively identify the key aspects of what happened.

3   Having clarified the key aspects, workshop attendees were then introduced to the concept of reflection as a means of turning experience into learning. To enable them to write a more formal reflective account, they were provided with reflective writing templates from professional organisations such as the Nursing and Midwifery Council and the General Medical Council, as well as an in-house version, which was adapted following consultation with allied health professional bodies. Time was provided to complete a formal reflective account that could then be submitted to support professional accreditation and revalidation, as evidence required at appraisals or for personal continuous professional development logs.

Evaluation of reflection for professional development training
Changes to the workshop were evaluated by using PDSA (plan, do, study, act) cycles to monitor improvements and data on session satisfaction was collected via course evaluation forms completed by attendees on the day. Findings included:

- The approach adapted well to various staff groups and worked successfully with a multi-disciplinary cohort, allowing for varying professional perspectives to shine new light on how an incident could be handled.
- Specific sessions with attendees from the same grade level or staff group would also be advantageous. The reasons behind this were unclear. One possibility is that higher grades of staff may wish to maintain their authoritative reputation, not feeling comfortable in 'opening up' to discuss incidents that might expose perceived weaknesses in a multi-disciplinary group.
- Differentiation in the need to evidence reflective practice for the appraisal system was highlighted as an area for further exploration. Higher grade staff, such as consultants, may need to format their writing to illustrate the application of reflective practice to patient care.
- Managers who first attended subsequently encouraged their team members to do likewise.
- Being provided with protected time and space to reflect on a deeper level and the facilitation of the processing of emotional experiences was valued by attendees.

When asked what participants found most useful, feedback included:

'Experiencing the wellbeing/psychological impact of reflection … letting people
know it may involve emotions – that's okay.' (Advanced Occupational
Therapist)

'Discussions around emotional response to workload … looking at frameworks.'
(Integrated Rehabilitation Team Manager)

'Session was conducted professionally and 1:1 was more focused/useful.'
(Consultant Psychiatrist)

'The reflective account activity as it really made me think in more detail about
the incident.' (HCA)

'Analysing situations and why they happened. What changes we can make.'
(Maternity apprentice)

'A relevant course for my studies. Found it very useful. It will be beneficial
when writing my future assignments.' (Trainee Operating Department
Practitioner)

Sticking points
Some reticence was expressed towards participating in the 'creative writing'
element – not all staff identify with being 'creative'. This prompted the
librarians to reframe the section as 'guided writing', making the activity less
daunting.

Due to the transportive element of the framework, participants were
advised not to revisit traumatic experiences to avoid triggering adverse
responses. The librarians were clear that they were not therapists and that the
sessions were not a debriefing intervention. Some managers felt that
addressing the emotional impact of incidents in this fashion was beneficial to
building resilience whilst enhancing the wellbeing offer of the organisation, so
would incorporate the tool into 1:1 debriefs with staff if needed.

Case study successes
In 2020, when working alongside COVID-19 began to negatively impact staff
within the Trust, the sessions were requested to support the wellbeing,
resilience and professionalism of both admin and clinical teams.

The successful redesign of the Reflective Practice training allowed staff to
look objectively at the key aspects of events to support professional
development and practice, turning experience into learning.

The exploration and reflection on the impact of challenging events
advanced the wellbeing strategies of both the Knowledge and Library Service
and the wider organisation.

There is potential that this approach could be successfully adopted widely, as exemplified through the rollout of the Holmes and Spencer workshops in various medical learning environments.

Key themes: creative writing, wellbeing, resilience, professionalism

Conclusion

In summary, reflective practice is a way of exploring a situation. It helps us to make meaning from our experiences and to develop opportunities for growth and improvement. While reflective practice is an approach that we use for individual learning and personal development, we can also use it to show how our services have developed. It helps us to think critically about the outcomes of our services and identify areas where we can make improvements. It enables us to pull together different strands of evidence into a narrative that will help us to make it clear to the validators what we do in support of each dimension and what steps we can take to make improvements.

Finally, in our roles as knowledge and library specialists, we can use the skills that we have developed as reflective practitioners to develop services to support healthcare professionals with their professional practice. We can provide access to resources, participate in group reflection and develop training and creative approaches for helping people to reflect.

References

Academy of Medical Royal Colleges/COPMeD (2018) *Reflective Practice Toolkit*. www.aomrc.org.uk/wp-content/uploads/2018/09/Reflective_ Practice_Toolkit_AoMRC_CoPMED_0818.pdf.

Bifarin, O. and Stonehouse, D. (2017) Clinical Supervision: An Important Part of Every Nurse's Practice, *British Journal of Nursing*, **26** (6), 331–5. www.magonlinelibrary.com/doi/pdf/10.12968/bjon.2017.26.6.331.

Borton, T. (1970) *Reach, Touch and Teach*, Hutchinson.

Care Quality Commission (CQC) (2018) *Quality Improvement in Hospital Trusts – Sharing Learning from Trusts on a Journey of QI*. www.cqc.org.uk/sites/default/files/20180911_QI_hospitals_FINAL.pdf.

CILIP (2020) *Chartership: Your Guide*. https://cdn.ymaws.com/www.cilip.org.uk/resource/resmgr/cilip_new_webs ite/professional_registration/mclip_guide_v1-0_20-11.pdf.

CIPD (2018) *What is Reflective Practice?* CIPD.

Clark, R. and McLean, C. (2018) The Professional and Personal Debriefing Needs of Ward Based Nurses After Involvement in a Cardiac Arrest: An Explorative Qualitative Pilot Study, *Intensive Crit Care Nursing*, **47**, 78– 84. https://pubmed.ncbi.nlm.nih.gov/29680586.

Collison, C. and Parcel, G. (2001) *Learning to Fly: Practical Knowledge Management from Leading and Learning Organizations*, Capstone.

General Medical Council (GMC) (2018) *New Guidance to Help you with Reflection*. www.gmc-uk.org/responsible-officer-hub/news/new-guidance-to-help-you-with-reflection.

General Medical Council (GMC) (2021) *The Reflective Practitioner – Guidance for Doctors and Medical Students*. www.gmc-uk.org/education/standards-guidance-and-curricula/guidance/reflective-practice/the-reflective-practitioner—-guidance-for-doctors-and-medical-students.

Gibbs, G. (1988) *Learning by Doing: A Guide to Teaching and Learning Methods*, Oxford Brookes University Further Education Unit.

Health and Care Professions Council (2021) *Reflective Practice*. www.hcpc-uk.org/standards/meeting-our-standards/reflective-practice.

Health Education England (2021) *Knowledge for Healthcare, Knowledge Mobilisation Toolkit: After Actions Review*s. https://library.hee.nhs.uk/knowledge-mobilisation/knowledge-mobilisation-toolkit/after-action-review.

Kolb, D. A. (1984) *Experiential Learning: Experience as the Source of Learning and Development (Vol. 1)*, Prentice-Hall.

Johns, C. (2017) *Becoming a Reflective Practitioner*, 5th edn, Wiley Blackwell.

Lucas, B. and Nacer, H. (2015) *The Habits of an Improver: Thinking About Learning For Improvement in Health Care*. The Health Foundation.

Miller, J. M., Ford, S. F. and Yang, A. (2020) Elevation Through Reflection: Closing the Circle to Improve Librarianship, *Journal of the Medical Library Association*, **108** (3), 353–63.

Milton, N. (2010) *The Lessons Learned Handbook: Practical Approaches to Learning From Experience*, Chandos Publishing.

Mindtools (2022) *STAR Method: A Model Approach to Nail Your Next Interview*. www.mindtools.com/pages/article/STAR-method.htm.

NHS England (2022) *Online Library of Quality, Service Improvement and Redesign Tools: Plan, Do, Study, Act (PDSA) Cycles and the Model for Improvement*. www.england.nhs.uk/wp-content/uploads/2022/01/qsir-pdsa-cycles-model-for-improvement.pdf.

Nursing and Midwifery Council (2018) *The Code: Professional Standards of Practice and Behaviour for Nurses, Midwives and Nursing Associates*. www.nmc.org.uk/standards/code.

Point of Care Foundation (2022) *About Schwartz Rounds*. www.pointofcarefoundation.org.uk/our-programmes/staff-experience/about-schwartz-rounds.

Royal College of Nursing (n.d.) *Revalidation Requirements: Reflection and Reflective Discussion.* www.rcn.org.uk/professional-development/revalidation/reflection-and-reflective-discussion.
Schon, D. (1991) *The Reflective Practitioner: How Professionals Think in Action*, Ashgate.

12

Looking to the Future of Healthcare Knowledge Services

Sue Lacey Bryant

Introduction

Prediction is very difficult, especially about the future.

Robert Storm Petersen (attrib.)

As knowledge specialists we are extraordinarily well placed to see what is before us, what is right in front of our eyes. As we shape the knowledge services of tomorrow, our professional responsibility is to move beyond what we can already discern as we use our information skills to examine the evidence, data and trends and look to action.

Demand for healthcare is rising rapidly everywhere (PWC, 2023) as the world's population is ageing. Every country in the world is experiencing growth in both the number and the proportion of older people. By 2030, 1 in 6 people will be aged 60 or over, an estimated 1.4 billion people worldwide. Between 2020 and 2050, the number of people aged 80 years or older is expected to triple to reach 426 million (World Health Organization (WHO), 2022).

Governments across the globe face growing pressure to reduce costs without limiting access to care and without impacting on quality. Hence, 'Health systems are optimising human resources and adopting process-driven advances, standardised procedures and technological innovations to cut costs and improve quality' (PWC, 2023).

Technological innovation is moving at pace, changing the nature of service delivery across sectors. People are familiar with applications from online shopping, social media and smart personal assistants to banking and travel. By 2015, Boeing 777 airline pilots were reporting that on a typical flight they spent a mere seven minutes manually flying the plane, primarily during take-off and landing (Markoff, 2015). Data privacy is a concern for many. However, users may be less aware of the risks of bias within the algorithms that lie behind these technologies.

The essential characteristics of high technology are newness and complexity. High technology operates near the frontier of knowledge.

(New Zealand Institute of Economic Research (NZIER), 2016, 5)

Healthcare is a knowledge intensive sector. Managing and applying knowledge – evidence from research and learning from experience – to better effect are part of the solution to the challenges identified. Investment in proactive knowledge services makes good business sense, impacting on quality, safety, productivity and cost.

The future of healthcare knowledge services is bright; it lies in the hands of our profession and it is important that we get it right.

The future of healthcare

Advances in the field of medicine are extraordinary, often nothing short of revolutionary. Published in 2019, the Topol Review observed that:

We are at a unique juncture in the history of medicine, with the convergence of genomics, biosensors, the electronic patient record and smartphone apps, all superimposed on a digital infrastructure, with artificial intelligence [AI] to make sense of the overwhelming amount of data created. This remarkably powerful set of information technologies provides the capacity to understand, from a medical standpoint, the uniqueness of each individual – and the promise to deliver healthcare on a far more rational, efficient and tailored basis.

(Topol, 2019, 6)

Inevitably, AI reflects the imperfections of its human developers. Citizens and healthcare staff must be alert to the risk that human biases may be built into predictive algorithms. People need knowledge and skills to critique AI-based tools, recognise biases and counteract them. The Topol Review highlighted that:

Capability must be developed … to identify and understand algorithmic bias and ensure that data does not reflect the bias inherent in social structures, and reinforce structural discrimination and inequalities.

(Topol, 2019, 11)

Automation bias, which leads clinicians to accept machine advice unquestion-ingly, poses further risks to patient safety. Training is needed to ensure they maintain vigilance and validate automated advice (Topol, 2019, 22).

COVID-19 has exacerbated pre-existing and 'ongoing challenges of health workforce deficits and imbalances' (WHO, 2020), shortened life expectancy and reversed progress in health improvement (United Nations (UN), 2022). Meanwhile, the WHO assesses climate change as the single biggest health threat facing humanity (WHO, 2021). Heatwaves, storms, floods, droughts and air pollution affect the social and environmental determinants of health – clean air, safe drinking water, sanitation, sufficient food and secure shelter – and they make it easier for diseases to spread across large groups of people (St George's University, 2021).

Within every region, political, economic and social factors may all impact on access to healthcare, driving health disparities. Inevitably, armed conflicts between warring states and groups present a serious challenge to universal healthcare, quickly destroying critical infrastructure, leaving people with non-communicable diseases without access to essential care, making everyone more vulnerable to diseases and impacting on mental health (St George's University, 2021).

Heart disease, stroke, cancer, respiratory diseases and diabetes account for 74% of all deaths globally. 77% of deaths from these chronic diseases, caused by a combination of genetic, physiological, environmental and behavioural factors, are in low- and middle-income countries (WHO, 2023). 'As people live longer, but also with more long-term conditions, there is an inexorable increase in the demand for healthcare' (Topol, 2019, 9).

Human resources are a major challenge too. Healthcare professionals are ageing and retiring; a shortage of skilled staff presents considerable challenges to health systems (PWC, 2023). With a vision of accelerating progress towards 'universal health coverage' by 2030, the WHO (2020) has long projected a shortfall of 18 million health workers by 2030, primarily in low- and lower-middle income countries.

In the face of these global challenges, health services cannot afford to be complacent. 'Affordability and efficiency is the future of healthcare' around the globe (Glass and Perkovic, 2021). It is crucial for patient safety and for hard-pressed systems to avoid waste as well as harm (Braithwaite, Glasziou and Westbrook, 2020).

> Healthcare represents a paradox. While change is everywhere, performance has flatlined: 60% of care on average is in line with evidence- or consensus-based guidelines, 30% is some form of waste or of low value, and 10% is harm. The 60-30-10 Challenge has persisted for three decades.
>
> (Braithwaite, Glasziou and Westbrook, 2020, 1)

Looking ahead, the optimum is for knowledge services to deploy knowledge specialists as part of the skill mix within healthcare teams to play a central role in reducing waste. This will allow organisations to improve productivity, release clinical time, enable practice to be more evidence-based and improve safety and care as well as reducing unnecessary or ineffective procedures.

The future healthcare workforce

The World Economic Forum (WEF) (Kearney, 2020) believes that four trends will shape the future of the healthcare workforce. As a small, highly specialised occupational group, each of these trends has implications for healthcare librarians and knowledge managers.

Firstly, non-clinical roles will become ever more important, crucial to support the whole patient (Kearney, 2020). This may translate into a wider range of social care, support and health coaching roles. The Topol Review (2019), which focused on preparing the healthcare workforce to deliver the digital future, anticipates new roles to address skills gaps in clinical bioinformatics, data analysts, digital technologists, AI and robotics and knowledge specialists (Topol, 2019).

Secondly, providers will prioritise reducing the administrative overhead. Currently, fragmented electronic health record systems add to the staff burden. The introduction of technology will change the composition of care teams and employees will increasingly leverage digital tools to increase their impact (Kearney, 2020). Examining the impact of technologies on the information professions, the CILIP *Technology Review* predicts that 'AI will replace repetitive forms of knowledge and service work, and robots will replace highly repetitive, predictable labour' (Cox, 2021, 11).

Thirdly, the scale of workforce shortages will drive employers to invest in attracting and retaining talent. Offering flexibility around working patterns and the potential for remote work via telehealth will each play a part. WEF expects to see proactive approaches to stress management and reducing workload to prevent burnout (Kearney, 2020). Library managers will want to look carefully at roles to determine the right balance between offering remote working and enabling face-to-face interaction with users and within their team.

Fourthly, the workforce of the future must be increasingly 'digital savvy'. There is an imperative to invest in capable, skilled health workers and reskilling and supporting employees in making the transition to deliver the digital future (Kearney, 2020).

Knowledge services have a particular role to play here in enabling digital inclusion and building the digital skills and confidence of staff and trainees, as well as enhancing their own knowledge and skills in using digital devices, applications and networks to create, manage and share digital content.

Almost all areas of the healthcare workforce will be affected over the next 20 years as digital technologies are adopted:

The pace of change will differ by speciality and by individual medical practice, but will ultimately impact on all healthcare professionals.

(Topol, 2018, 21)

We can anticipate a gradual, yet substantial, reconfiguration of clinical roles accompanied by acceleration of the shift towards multi-disciplinary working. 'Roles will become more fluid; role boundaries may blur' (Topol, 2019, 68).

As already noted, AI will be applied to undertake repetitive tasks within knowledge services. However, information professionals can expect that digital technologies 'will also create many jobs' for people to develop tools and undertake analysis and for domain experts (Cox, 2021, 11).

How far will technological change address the workforce supply challenge? The evidence suggests that new technologies will primarily slow down the growth of employment in healthcare rather than reduce it (Bronsoler, Doyle and Van Reenen, 2020). The Topol Review (2019) concluded that 'technologies will not replace healthcare professionals, but will enhance them ("augment them"), giving them more time to care for patients' (Topol, 2019, 9).

Skills for the future

How to keep up with the future of work? The answer is to skill, re-skill and re-skill again (World Economic Forum, 2017).

The McKinsey Global Institute predicts that in the future world of work, and irrespective of occupation and sector, everyone in the labour market will need to meet three criteria: (1) add value beyond what can be done by automated systems and intelligent machines; (2) operate in a digital environment; and (3) continually adapt to new ways of working and new occupations (McKinsey and Company, 2021). It has been estimated that the half-life of a learned skill is 5 years (Gibson, 2015). This means that much of what health librarians learned 10 years ago is already obsolete and half of what we learned 5 years ago is irrelevant. To future-proof careers, clinicians and knowledge specialists alike need to keep ahead of the curve and start learning new skills sooner rather than later. Preparing for the future, individuals may want to self-assess their skills within the four broad categories identified by McKinsey and Company (2021), which identified 56 foundational skills in all:

1 Cognitive skills, encompassing critical thinking, planning and ways of working, communication and mental flexibility – which includes translating knowledge to different contexts.
2 Interpersonal skills including mobilising systems, developing relationships, teamwork effectiveness.

3 Self-leadership requiring self-awareness and self-management, entrepreneurship, goals achievement.
4 Foundational digital skills including digital fluency and citizenship, software use and development, understanding digital systems – which incorporates digital literacy, data privacy and cyber-security literacy.

Information mastery remains crucial for the clinicians of today and tomorrow (Hutchinson et al., 2012). The volume of scientific knowledge is expanding exponentially meaning that the workforce has to contend with an extraordinary degree of information overload. Estimates indicate that medical knowledge doubled every seven years in 1980, every three and a half years by 2010 and that by 2020 it would double every 73 days (Densen, 2011). Maggio and Artino (2018, 597) believe that while they could help battle information overload, 'librarians are an underutilized resource'.

Information overload outstrips the information processing capacity of the brain. Doctors 'experience a higher background level of anxiety at work because of concerns about giving poor advice or forgetting something important because of the volume of information they are trying to process' (Sbaffi et al., 2020). While 'physicians must remain current (i.e., *the informed physician*) and follow the policies and directives reported in the guidelines to guarantee the quality of patient care … the pressure of being up to date and making sure nothing is overlooked plays a considerable role in increasing physicians' stress' (Sbaffi et al., 2020).

Part of the mission of the knowledge services of the future is surely to mitigate the information stress felt by healthcare staff? Clinicians can no longer keep on top of this pace of change without the right decision support tools, without digital as a driver or without proactive knowledge services delivered by specialised librarians and knowledge managers.

Priorities for healthcare knowledge services in the future

As the human bridge between knowledge sources and knowledge users, the healthcare knowledge specialists of tomorrow will play a central role in the health and care knowledge economy, just as they do today. See Figure 12.1 opposite.

To design the health knowledge services of the future requires a determined focus on purpose. It is a 'given' that the role and functions of health knowledge services must be driven by a close understanding of organisational challenges, needs and priorities. This extends beyond what paymasters and users say they want. Rather, it is imperative that service managers convey to executive teams the full potential of appropriately

Main stakeholders in the health and care knowledge economy

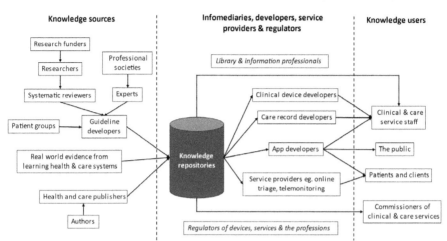

Figure 12.1 *Main stakeholders in the health and care knowledge economy.*
By permission of Jeremy Wyatt, University of Southampton.

resourced health knowledge services as part of the solution to the challenges that health systems face.

Great customer care is always at the heart of knowledge service delivery, whether that is face-to-face or working on digital products for health professionals to use. It is our knowledge of customers and potential customers that will underpin successful health knowledge services. Truly knowing customers and their preferences, appreciating their priorities and the challenges they face, and understanding the knowledge needs of different occupational groups through different stages of their career will inform service redesign.

Supporting education, practice, research and innovation will remain central. However, the relative balance of knowledge service delivery towards each purpose, the nature of those knowledge services, the shape of the workforce and ways of working, will all transform over the next 15 years.

Over the coming years, we can anticipate higher priority being given to:

- embedded librarianship
- knowledge manager roles and functions
- teaching information skills
- knowledge mobilisation techniques
- facilitating the adoption of proven innovations
- nurturing health learning systems
- improving health and digital literacy skills.

Clinical decision support systems are an essential feature of future knowledge service provision. See the section on 'decision support' below.

The challenges and the opportunities will vary from country to country, and from setting to setting, and the speed of transformation will vary too. Nevertheless, now is the time to revisit priorities and explore new opportunities. Today's service managers will want to foster an environment in which experimentation is encouraged and apply the learning to prepare for possible futures.

Managers will also need to determine the optimum scale of operation to make the most of opportunities to expand and extend knowledge service provision, optimise specialist skills and yield the benefits of automation to achieve economies of scale. As a result, some services will want to enter into a more formal partnership, or amalgamate, to better serve a larger geographical footprint or a group of clinical specialities. Figure 12.2 indicates criteria to inform service redesign (Health Education England, 2021a, 61).

Nationwide functions	Function will benefit from national leadership to achieve delivery across England
Specialist skills	Function requires scarce specialist skills which may not be accessible across the country
Economy of scale	Function can generate economics of scale, offering value for money if delivered at a larger scale
Opportunity for standardisation	Function can be delivered using a standardised approach across a wider region or customer base
Local knowledge	Function requires in-depth knowledge of the needs of the local economy and active partnership working

Figure 12.2 *Criteria for the redesign of knowledge and library services*

Embedded roles

CILIP published a Corporate Library and Information Services Survey in 2018 (McDonald, 2018). This reported increasing demand, across sectors, for 'decision-ready information' accompanied by a trend towards increasingly becoming an embedded profession (McDonald, 2018).

The expectation is that healthcare knowledge and library services will see growing demand for knowledge specialists embedded within clinical and management teams (Health Education England, 2015). Already 81% of the knowledge services that are funded by the NHS in England offer clinical, outreach or embedded librarian services – occupying 26% of knowledge service staff time (Health Education England, 2021b).

> Aligned to multidisciplinary teams, embedded knowledge specialists release the time of health professionals by seeking out evidence and good practice.
>
> (Health Education England, 2021a, 25)

Clinical librarians provide a valuable service that impacts on direct patient care, improves quality and saves money within healthcare organisations (Brettle, Maden and Payne, 2016). Hence, 'the future is bright for that mix of expert searching skills, communication, organisational skills and confidence to proactively promote and market health and social care information resources' (NcNally, 2021).

Research in the critical care unit of one teaching hospital showed a wide range of benefits. The embedded clinical librarian role 'helped staff to learn, develop and improve the quality of their care. It nurtured an evidence-based culture across the department and generated a positive financial value from saving staff time, supporting their professional development and improving patient care (Sadera, 2019, 8). Further, a health economics study in 2020 found that key features of a high performing NHS library service included 'specialty/departmental alignment, preferably with embedded knowledge specialists' (Economics by Design, 2020, 11).

With close knowledge of the priorities of the healthcare teams to which they are aligned, embedded knowledge specialists are well placed to deliver targeted and tailored alerts. The production of bulletins and alerting services is but one example of service delivery for which the healthcare knowledge services of the future will be more impactful where they collaborate across a larger footprint, geographically and nationally. Working together, and streamlining processes, will extend the reach of targeted and tailored information products to better address the pressure on clinicians to remain up to date in their field.

Knowledge management

Knowledge and information can be seen as the currency of successful healthcare organisations (Health Education England, 2021a). Using research evidence, implementing best practice and innovation, and sharing hard-won learning from experience are all business critical. The Topol Review urged executive boards of NHS organisations to take responsibility for effective knowledge management to strengthen systems to disseminate learning and accelerate adoption of proven technological innovations (Topol, 2019).

The successful knowledge specialists of tomorrow will develop new tools to assess how well the organisation is managing and deploying corporate knowledge, using evidence from research and harnessing the knowledge of the workforce to inform policy and practice. They will use technology to curate, mine and apply organisational knowledge as an asset (see Chapter 5 for a discussion of how knowledge and evidence is currently 'mobilised').

Growing demand can be anticipated not only for embedded knowledge brokers, responsible for searching and presenting evidence that is synthesised and summarised, but also for knowledge managers who can marshal corporate knowledge and staff know-how to underpin strategy and operations (Health Education England, 2021a). While in health services 'It should be everyone's job to create, share, and use knowledge to some degree' (Davenport, 1997), in future, facilitating knowledge exchange and mobilising staff know-how, within and across healthcare organisations, networks and systems, will be a larger role for health knowledge services.

Information literacy

Alongside promoting the use of evidence, librarians have a role in educating healthcare professionals to find the best evidence for their purpose and to be confident to question that evidence.

Widespread use of clinical decision support, and the intuitive discovery systems of the future, will allow novice searchers to access information readily. This will not negate their need to understand: how to frame a clinical question; the methodology that underpins an effective literature search; and the potential biases within the body of research and within the machine learning (ML) powered tools they may be using to filter their search results. Helping healthcare workers acquire these critical information skills is core business for health knowledge services. Partly due to the time pressures on clinical staff, perhaps also to growing appreciation of the expertise of information professionals, 'the role of health care librarians has evolved in recent years, leading to greater demand for their involvement in supporting the critical appraisal of evidence and its subsequent uptake' (Sabey and Biddle, 2021, 434).

Technological advances will offer fresh opportunities in the future to explore how simulation, 3D virtual environments and game-based learning can be used to engage clinicians in information skills training (Ou, Felicia and Kane, 2013). There may be opportunities here to help trainees, in particular, use 'time confetti' to good purpose by providing 'just in time' information to build both knowledge and information literacy skills (Wickramarachchi, 2021).

Spread and adoption of innovation

In future, knowledge specialists can play an important role not only in bringing evidence to the fore, but also in raising awareness amongst healthcare staff of models, tools and techniques of spread, adoption and implementation of innovation.

A key principle set by the Topol Review was that 'the adoption of digital healthcare technologies should be grounded in compelling real-world evidence of clinical efficacy and cost-effectiveness, followed by practical knowledge transfer throughout the NHS' (Topol, 2019, 200). Accordingly, there is an urgent need for knowledge specialists to double their efforts to incorporate the evaluation of innovations, including technological innovations, into their training offer and to advise on implementation models that simply presume that the value of an intervention is already proven.

> The transformational benefits that innovations in science and technology, such as artificial intelligence, can bring for patients and staff require a shift to a lifelong learning mindset throughout the NHS.
>
> (Topol, 2019, 800)

The Topol Review argues that everyone must be supported to develop the mindset, skill set and behaviours that will empower the workforce of the future (Topol, 2019).

Learning health systems

Real, sustainable, active improvement of healthcare over time depends on a 'culture of continual learning that helps everyone to grow' (Berwick, 2013, 44). There is growing interest around the world in the emerging concept of 'learning health systems'. Librarians have key roles to play in this future, including in pinpointing information needs and gaps and assisting health services to optimise the use of knowledge and evidence for decision making (Walker, 2018, 38).

> A Learning Health System can improve the use of research evidence, staff knowhow, learning from experience and organisational memory. It can close the loop by delivering knowledge back to the front-line, in a form that is likely to be acted upon.
>
> (Foley, Horwitz and Zahran, 2021, 11)

An organisational culture that rewards knowledge sharing rather than knowledge hoarding and individual commitment to continuous learning is a critical factor in learning health systems. Healthcare knowledge services will continue to play a pivotal role in nurturing a learning culture as well as in supporting individual learners, not simply in their early years of training but through continuing professional development.

Health knowledge specialists also have a vital role to play in building a learning culture and empowering clinicians with the skills and confidence to use evidence sources with peers, teams and patients.

Equally, higher education institutions play a fundamental role in building the curious, agile and flexible healthcare workforce of the future by imparting information skills for lifelong learning and helping learners bridge the gap between academe and practice. Academic library teams need to be familiar with the knowledge sources and tools likely to be available to their alumni as they become practitioners. Ever closer liaison between academic librarians and knowledge specialists in healthcare organisations will help trainees transition so that they can continue to draw on the knowledge they need just in time.

Health and digital literacy

Health literacy is about people having enough knowledge, understanding, skills and confidence to use health information, to be active partners in their care, and to navigate health and social care systems.

(Carlyle et al., 2023)

Limited health literacy levels are associated with poorer self-management skills, poorer health outcomes, and increased health care use.

(van der Gaag et al., 2022, 2)

The trend towards digital-first health services is set to continue, with patients asked to use online consultation systems, as well as book appointments online, and more health information being published online only (Carlyle, 2022). This calls for the public, patients, families and carers to have both digital skills and health literacy skills. There is an urgent need to equip people to navigate the healthcare system, to find information and to differentiate between fact and fallacy, so that they can use health information for self-care and shared decision-making. The dangers of misinformation and disinformation were highlighted through the experience of the pandemic, and the associated infodemic, as discussed in Chapter 7.

Given rising demand for healthcare (PWC, 2023), these skills are increasingly important to the affordability and sustainability of health services into the future. In the years ahead, governments and healthcare provider organisations can be expected to place increasing emphasis on enabling people to engage with digital health services productively and safely. Similarly, as part of broader initiatives to address health inequalities, there will be a renewed focus on raising levels of health literacy to help individuals use health information to make choices (Department of Health and Social Care, 2021).

Drawing on their expert knowledge of health information sources and how to evaluate these, health knowledge specialists will make a valuable contribution by training other librarians and information providers within their communities. Strong partnership working skills will be needed to shape sustainable local initiatives using an asset-based strategy.

The healthcare workforce needs to be fluent in health literacy and also agile in adapting to new digital products. 'The development of information skills and information literacy resonate with the need for explainable AI' (Cox, 2021, 31). Nor are healthcare staff immune from digital poverty and, for some years to come, connectivity will remain challenging in some geographies. Therefore, the role for knowledge services in upskilling healthcare staff and providing access to online facilities remains into the future.

Knowledge specialists can be expected to look to technology-enhanced learning to produce engaging learning resources for professionals and for citizens.

AI-powered knowledge services for the future

The essential 'ask' of clinicians to maintain their knowledge is extraordinary. In the UK, as an example, nurses and midwives are required to always practise in line with the best available evidence and to keep the knowledge and skills they need for safe and effective practice up to date (Nursing and Midwifery Council (NMC), 2018). Similarly, doctors must be familiar with guidelines and developments that affect their work and provide effective treatments based on the best available evidence (General Medical Council, 2023). To enable practitioners to meet these high standards, librarians will want to explore the potential of AI and ML in particular to reimagine information products, knowledge management tools and knowledge services.

'AI and robots are our past, present and future' (Cox, 2021, 8). These are exciting times as AI and ML open the door to new opportunities to unlock the value of evidence from research. Crucially, to quote Andrew Cox, 'the information, knowledge management and library workforce has opportunities, and an important role in choosing about the collective future, through how it responds to the current wave of technologies' (Cox, 2021, 11).

Published in 2021, CILIP research showed that ideas about AI, ML, process automation and robotics were already changing the ways in which users interact with information (Cox, 2021). The review found that 'there are changes happening across the whole information value chain: in its production, organisation and consumption' (Cox, 2021, 3).

This is a time of experimentation in how healthcare staff and learners might benefit from AI applications. Health librarians in England, for example, have reported on initiatives using AI to support new information-seeking behaviours and improve the search experience, including to help researchers construct complex searches, and also on developing knowledge services by introducing chatbots (Health Education England, 2021c).

AI in resource discovery

The most obvious application of AI is to discovery systems. We can expect extraordinary changes in the provision of knowledge services over the next 15 to 20 years, partly shaped by advances in knowledge management solutions on the market. Perhaps 'the most important application of AI arises from the way it creates potential for information services to support new ways to analyse content' (Cox, 2021, 19). A shift 'from the paradigm of searching for items to read manually to the model of extracting knowledge from collections of text, images and other data through algorithms' (Cox, 2021, 3) is sometimes presented as a binary choice. Surely the two models will co-exist, with healthcare knowledge services of the future facilitating the former, especially to support particular forms of learning, and the latter to deliver knowledge content as close as possible to the point of care?

Knowledge discovery systems are becoming increasingly sophisticated, incorporating AI, natural language processing (NLP) and taxonomies to enhance search functionality, return more relevant results and improve the user experience. Vendors will continue to develop new tools to enrich the discovery process, helping researchers to explore content, trialling new approaches in comparison with conventional expert searching. Knowledge graphs can open up new lines of enquiry by enabling researchers to visualise the relationship between concepts.

In the future, healthcare knowledge specialists are likely to be involved in supporting a mix of discovery services and knowledge management products to help healthcare professionals surface the knowledge they need. Figure 12.3 opposite, taken from the CILIP Review, illustrates different forms of socio-technical infrastructure that may be put in place across a health economy, or nationally, to support knowledge discovery (Cox, 2021).

The CILIP Review notes that changes 'to web and mobile search imply a need for what has been called algorithmic literacy, as an aspect of information literacy' (Cox, 2021, 4).

Health librarians of the future will want to be well positioned to critique information products and knowledge management tools to aid selection and inform the training of healthcare professionals and learners. Part of the wider support service role will surely be to ensure that users understand that search engines are driven by commercial motives; that there are layers of network bias in how search results are produced and presented; that these are affected by data voids, keyword appropriation, filter bubbles, echo chambers, deep

	Content	Technical infrastructure	Information service role
1 A projects-specific assembly of digital content and tools	Temporary, researcher chosen	Temporary, ad-hoc	Background support
2 A local content collection, such as a know-how collection in a law firm	Locally developed, unpublished content	Permanent	Assembling content, training tools, supporting usage
3 Digitised or born digital content in the special collections of a research library	Locally unpublished content, often digitised	Temporary for each project	Providing content, supporting usage
4 A sector wide aggregation of content available for mining	Published content	Collective	Signposting the service to users
5 A tool/content agnostic infrastructure within which bespoke collections of content for different types of analysis are stored	Any	For storage and tools	Building and promoting infrastructure
6 A publisher or aggregator platform including content and tools — subscribed to by an information service for users	Publisher owned or aggregated	Licensed	Licensing service and supporting use
7 A semi-permanent assembly of content, infrastructure, tools and people for a very specific, ongoing purpose, such as in a living systematic review	Information service selected from published sources	Semi-permanent	Controlling an integrated solution
8 A support service that focuses on advice on tools, training and supporting collaboration	None	Human rather than technical	Assembling expertise and building community

Figure 12.3 *Alternatives of socio-technical infrastructures to support AI in knowledge discovery*

fakes, automated content moderation and more; and, not least, that confirmation bias and unconscious bias impact information-seeking behaviours (Cox, 2021, 18).

Decision support

Clinical decision support systems, which augment the work of clinicians in a variety of decisions and tasks, are a good exemplar of how healthcare professionals may experience the application of new technology to knowledge solutions in the future.

Getting computers to do tasks that would usually require human intelligence, AI and ML (allowing computer systems to learn from examples) have great potential to improve diagnosis, treatment and prognosis of a particular medical condition. Bringing real-time clinical data gathered from medical devices and records together with the evidence base is expected to enable precise and relevant predictions:

A growing number of artificial intelligence (AI)-based clinical decision support systems are showing promising performance in preclinical, in silico, evaluation, but few have yet demonstrated real benefit to patient care.

(Vasey et al., 2022, 1)

Nevertheless, use of decision support is a practical priority 'to help clinicians in applying best practice, eliminate unwarranted variation across the whole pathway of care' (NHS England, 2019, 92).

These tools play into wider knowledge service initiatives to drive a culture of learning and evidence-based practice. Decision support is all about knowledge translation, intended to improve healthcare delivery by targeting clinical knowledge, patient information and other health information to enhance medical decisions (Sutton et al., 2020). On the downside, clinicians fear such tools generate unnecessary alerts, causing information stress, and result in alarm fatigue, leading to worse outcomes (Sutton et al., 2020). Therefore, health librarians will want to get involved in the selection, procurement, implementation and marketing of clinical decision support systems. Bringing critical evaluation skills into play, knowledge specialists can take a key role in helping healthcare professionals understand the pros and cons of different products on the market and assess options for integration into the electronic health record to best deliver knowledge to the frontline.

Clinical guidelines

Decision support tools will continue to draw on clinical practice *guidance* as well as the latest evidence-based research and expert opinion. Performing systematic reviews is time-consuming and resource-intensive. Moreover, the sheer volume of scientific publishing adds to the pressures on national bodies charged to develop clinical guidance. In the coming years, this challenge seems likely to prompt further experimentation with text mining and analytical products aimed at reducing the time needed to screen search results and speed up the systematic review process (Yamada et al., 2020).

From a strategic perspective, will national bodies continue to invest in developing guidance across the broad spectrum of clinical topics? Or will they instead focus resources on high priority areas, those conditions that drive the majority of healthcare utilisation for which guidance may add the greatest value? The latter would potentially generate new demand on local healthcare knowledge services, either in the form of requests for rapid reviews to answer immediate questions about patient care or requests for systematic reviews to inform local guidance on less common conditions. Both will generate demands on the time and skill set of healthcare knowledge specialists.

In this evolving landscape, future knowledge specialists will want to differentiate between the skills of the general searcher and their own expertise, demarcating the added value they deliver by deploying advanced search strategies and filtering and through summarising and synthesising just enough evidence for healthcare teams to use in their work.

Evidence summaries

This is a time of experimentation in how healthcare staff and learners might benefit from AI applications. Health librarians in England, for example, have reported on initiatives using AI to improve the search experience, to help researchers construct complex searches (Health Education England, 2021c).

One service describes a fully automated evidence synthesis tool for identifying, assessing and collating the evidence. It shows that ML, NLP, rule-based systems and modern visualisation techniques can be used to identify, assess and collate research findings to produce evidence maps, which points to time savings in synthesising evidence (Brassey et al., 2021).

Certainly, there may be benefits in expanding the menu of outputs of systematic searches, for example, presenting evidence maps in a user-friendly format to inform policy reviews.

It is already clear that the knowledge services of tomorrow will capitalise on AI, ML and NLP to augment the work of human searchers, enhancing the efficiency of evidence sifting and synthesis. For the foreseeable future, rather than replacing the work of knowledge specialists, extensive human validation will still be required (Blaizot et al., 2022).

Interacting with users

Taking a cue from commercial websites, chatbot systems that are programmed using conversational AI technology to simulate human conversation through text interfaces will offer new ways to interact with users. We can expect to welcome the chatbot to the healthcare knowledge service team of the future, partly to meet users' expectations of 24/7 digital services and partly to release staff time to deliver higher value services, such as tailored alerting services for executive teams, participating in clinical team reviews of treatment options or facilitating an after-action review. Chatbots can be used to automate routine customer enquiries and link users into discovery services and clinical decision support, as appropriate (Cox, 2021). Requiring investment upfront, not least in the time of an information professional to build the knowledge base for the chatbot, it may be more economic to develop and operate these applications across a network of libraries to serve a wider customer base group. Equally, highly specialised solo health libraries may yield benefit from introducing one, expanding capacity to support clients.

The CILIP Review discusses the smart library concept in which sensors could be used 'to nudge behaviour, such as to encourage users who have not moved for a long time to take a break, for their well-being' (Cox, 2021, 25). This concept is perhaps more applicable to academic libraries than the knowledge and learning hub spaces that we might expect to see available for practitioners within healthcare facilities.

Jobs

Will healthcare knowledge specialists lose jobs to the new technologies? The CILIP Review concludes that 'AI and robots will create, change and destroy jobs' (Cox, 2021, 10).

Some repetitive roles will become obsolete, replaced by robotic process automation (RPA), and that time can be freed up by the adoption of new technologies. Forward-looking service leads will be focusing on talent management now, actively developing the talent of paraprofessional staff through role expansion, for instance as health and digital skills trainers, and supporting career advancement through further study, for instance to gain qualifications in information science, knowledge management or health informatics.

In the short to medium term, AI-driven knowledge management solutions will augment the work of human knowledge specialists. There is a potential risk of disintermediation over time should it prove possible to use AI and robots on more complex tasks, including those seemingly requiring expert judgement and empathy (Cox, 2021).

However, in healthcare, AI and ML are already reshaping the ways that healthcare teams 'create, discover, use and share information' (Health Education England, 2021a, 49). Accordingly, this is not a time for doomsayers but, rather, one for those with a clear sense of purpose in bringing knowledge to healthcare and a willingness to adapt and adopt new ways of working. New priorities are emerging for knowledge services. As a result, we can expect to see new roles such as for knowledge architects, taxonomists, UX (user experience) librarians, research data management librarians and data visualisation librarians. Systems librarians are likely to see an expanded range of responsibilities and, similarly, the role of patient information specialists may be extended.

Competencies for the future

The CILIP Review found that the great strength of information professionals in responding to the future opportunities afforded by AI is the strong alignment between our existing skill set and the demands of new technologies (Cox, 2021).

Knowledge service teams are experienced in organising knowledge, knowledge architecture, collections management and copyright, metadata, information management and retrieval, procurement and licensing knowledge resources. Health knowledge services of the future will be hungry for these skills and there will also be new opportunities for librarians as technologists.

Librarians are trusted (Ipsos MORI, 2021a), respected and can draw on user support. So-called 'soft skills' seem set to become even more important in future and these are the ones at which computers will remain poor. Health librarians build on a track record of collaboration, within regional networks and both nationally and internationally.

Empathy and excellent communication skills lie at the heart of the reference interview and are crucial to the ability to synthesise and summarise evidence. Persuasion, influencing and negotiating are all-important for working across organisational boundaries and are important strengths for procurement.

The CILIP Review anticipates a huge opportunity for the information professions to position ourselves as trusted information professionals holding a range of roles, including offering authoritative support into our organisations and to staff and learners on how to harness these technologies while minimising the risks (Cox, 2021).

'Data-driven technologies offer great potential for the delivery of health and care in general and may have a specific part to play in helping to reduce disparities in health' (O'Brien et al., n.d., 6). However, there is also a risk that AI technologies may exacerbate existing health inequities for minority ethnic groups (O'Brien et al., n.d.). Indeed, the Topol Review identified that knowledge and skills in 'critical appraisal of digital healthcare technologies – understanding how the technology works, including the statistics underpinning machine learning and its outputs, and the potential biases' is essential learning for the whole healthcare workforce (Topol, 2019, 54).

Critical evaluation skills, and teaching critical appraisal, are already a strong feature of health librarianship. Identifying inherent bias and understanding limitations within evidence, and also within search functionality and reporting, are all an extension of the existing skill set of information professionals. There may well be a role for future health information professionals to step into the space of equipping commissioners and procurement teams to critique health products as part of their selection processes.

Meanwhile, as the dangers of 'fake news' become better understood, some groups will place greater value on human assistance from information professionals as a trusted source of information. See Chapter 6 for an exploration of this issue.

While CILIP found uncertainty among information professionals in many sectors, it reported that 'the lack of vision is not universal. One exception to this picture seems to be the health sector, where the NHS is seeing its future as very much digital' (Cox, 2021, 28). Indeed, the Topol Review proposed that to prepare for the digital future, all healthcare professionals need to be trained in health data provenance, curation, integration and governance; the ethics of AI and autonomous systems/tools; and the critical appraisal and interpretation of AI and robotics technologies (Topol, 2019). Knowledge specialists clearly have much to offer in this space as we move into the future.

Identifying skill gaps

Health informatics, the intelligent use of data and technology to improve patient safety and the quality of care, will help to shape the future of healthcare delivery. 'Big data' is of increasing importance in the health sector as health systems hold vast repositories of data that could be analysed computationally to reveal patterns, trends and links. The CILIP Review identified a need for knowledge specialists to gain a deeper understanding of computational thinking (Cox, 2021). There will be a growing requirement for greater fluency with computational systems and the mathematical and statistical techniques needed for the accurate analysis and interpretation of data. The research anticipates the importance of information professionals being confident in incremental tailoring and combining of applications to meet evolving needs, seeing applications as ongoing, co-designed artefacts rather than 'technological givens' (Cox, 2021).

Data science, which involves applying advanced analytics to extract valuable information from data, and data stewardship (data management and governance on behalf of healthcare organisations) will become more prominent (Cox, 2021). Moving into the future, health knowledge specialists can build on their portable knowledge: transferring into new contexts an understanding of the provenance of content, its limitations and potential bias; applying skills in subject description, categorisation and taxonomies; and all underpinned by a commitment to standards, unique identifiers and interoperability.

To support all the ways in which AI can be harnessed to surface content in future, knowledge specialists will want to be at the forefront of developing and offering training in algorithmic literacy for healthcare professionals and citizens (Cox, 2021). Algorithmic literacy will need to be embraced as a subset of information literacy skills to ensure healthcare professionals and citizens are alive to the limitations and influences of search engine bias and better able to critically evaluate search results. The same applies to teaching personal data privacy as an element of digital skills to underpin health literacy.

However, future skills requirements are far from being all about digital technology. 'Fusion skills' will be highly valued and crucial to enabling organisations to bring the machine into the team to rehumanise time, releasing headspace for decision-making and capacity for health knowledge specialists to build interpersonal connections and engage with clinical teams. Additionally, 'relentless reimagining' will be needed, emphasising the need to transform processes rather than automate existing ones (Daugherty and Wilson, 2018).

Professional knowledge and skills for the future

Forward-looking individuals investing in their own professional future now will find it helpful to reflect on their current skill set and to nurture their personal professional development. Using a skills or competencies framework can be a very helpful tool to expand thinking.

In the UK, the CILIP Professional Knowledge Skills Base (PKSB) is the sector skills standard for the information, knowledge, library and data profession (see Figure 12.4). The PKSB is freely available to all NHS knowledge and library staff in England through a partnership agreement between Health Education England and CILIP (CILIP, 2021). Recognising the imperative for health knowledge specialists to prepare for the future, Health Education England sponsored the revision of the PKSB in 2021, partly in the light of the CILIP Technology Review. New sections about data management and knowledge management were incorporated (Gilroy, 2021).

Health Education England co-produced healthcare sector guidance notes to help NHS knowledge and library specialists maximise the benefits of using the PKSB as a career development tool. The guidance offers practical examples of how knowledge and skills may apply to roles in health knowledge services (Gilroy, 2021).

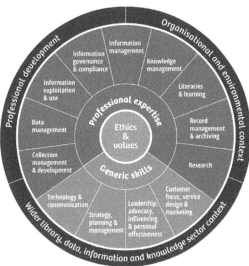

Figure 12.4 *The CILIP Professional Knowledge and Skills Base (PKSB)*

Ethics

Ethics and values lie at the heart of the PKSB.

The Topol Review anticipated a need for all healthcare professionals to be educated and trained in 'health data provenance, curation, integration and governance; the ethics of AI and autonomous systems/tools; and the critical appraisal and statistical interpretation of AI and robotics technologies' (Topol, 2019, 56).

'Librarianship is, in its very essence, an ethical activity embodying a value-rich approach to professional work with information', declares the International Federation of Library Associations and Institutions (IFLA) *Code of Ethics for Librarians and Other Information Workers* (IFLA, 2012, 1). The information profession 'has an important role to play in foregrounding ethical issues and finding ethical and safe ways to use AI and robots for the benefit of society' (Topol, 2019, 31).

Research skills

The adoption of evidence-based practices is dependent on robust research into library and information science. Research skills are important to the future of health knowledge services. While research is important across the sector, several areas stand out as requiring collective effort: evaluating technological solutions; the implications of AI bias in discovery tools; assessing return on investment in knowledge management functions; testing different methods of upskilling people in digital and health literacy skills; and, not least, strengthening the value proposition for the work of health knowledge and library specialists.

Ongoing financial pressures can be predicted. The International Monetary Fund notes that 'limited fiscal space for raising health spending" focuses the attention of policymakers "on ensuring that resources are used efficiently" (International Monetary fund (IMF), 2022). Clinicians and managers, including knowledge service managers, are therefore fortunate to be able to draw on a growing and consistent body of robust international evidence that investment in proactive knowledge services yields a sound return on investment, generating a cost benefit ratio of 1:2:4 by providing time-saving accelerated access to better quality evidence. This, in turn, enables staff to utilise evidence from research, and releases their time so they can use it more effectively (IFLA, 2020).

Significantly, a health economic analysis conducted in England further demonstrated that this 'gift of time' to clinicians (discussed throughout this book) does not take account of 'the wider value of improved access to higher quality evidence and the impact this has on patient outcomes and experience, operational efficiency and workforce development' (Economics by Design,

2020, 19). One study reports an overall benefit cost ratio of 3:1 once the wider benefits for staff and patients are incorporated (Brettle, Maden and Payne, 2016).

Health Education England completed another analysis illustrating that NHS libraries with better staff ratios are more able to work proactively with a wider range of healthcare teams to enable evidence-based decision-making. This has a positive impact on treatment options and the quality of patient care as well as impacting on productivity gains and cost improvement and the spread of innovation (NHS Library and Knowledge Services in England, 2020).

Together, these studies position knowledge services to advocate for greater investment. As an example, Health Education England has introduced a policy recommending that NHS organisations improve the staff ratio for the number of qualified library and knowledge specialists per member of the health workforce and also optimise the benefits of embedded and knowledge management roles (NHS Library and Knowledge Services in England, 2020).

To achieve the benefits that mobilising knowledge can bring to healthcare, and to secure sustainable funding for library and knowledge services, information professionals will need to build and use compelling evidence. As today, tomorrow's knowledge service managers will be wise to embed capturing impact data within business-as-usual in order to be able to demonstrate the value of knowledge services and their impact on health outcomes, productivity and economic benefit.

Advocacy and influencing

Leadership, advocacy (discussed in Chapter 4), influencing and personal effectiveness are also noteworthy in their own right as essential competencies for the future.

Harnessing persuasive data to achieve a high profile, demonstrating the different types of value that knowledge services add, is the work of good times as well as preparation for any future scenarios that bring services under scrutiny. Advocacy, recruiting influential champions and crafting a persuasive narrative will underpin the success of the knowledge services of the future. Perception is everything. Already familiar with contesting the illusion that there is 'free access' to sound evidence via the internet, it is not enough for librarians to be among the most trusted professions, second only to nurses – and ahead of doctors, in third place (Ipsos MORI, 2021b).

In a survey of sources that physicians find most useful when in need of medical information, the top four are: local clinical guidelines; national clinical guidelines; colleagues; and evidence-based practice. 'Librarians' ranked ninth out of ten (Sbaffi et al., 2020). It is critical for success that health librarians make visible the roles we play in developing and curating guidelines; keeping colleagues updated; and delivering the tools, sources, skills and synthesising and summarising services that underpin evidence-based practice.

Now is the time to influence executive boards, recruit champions, test thinking and set priorities for the health knowledge services of the future.

Career pathways

Given the trend towards more embedded, team-based professional roles (Health Education England, 2021a) and the potential to apply RPA to automate repetitive tasks, the profile of the health knowledge services workforce is set to change (Health Education England, 2021c). Over time, it will morph from the current pyramid in which most jobs are held by paraprofessional and junior staff, with very few senior posts. The future workforce will assume the shape of a diamond in which the majority of posts are for professionally qualified knowledge specialists, with far fewer paraprofessional support staff. While there will be relatively few senior roles, there will be new and wider vistas to be explored, as well as opportunities for knowledge specialists to move into more strategic roles.

Direct experience indicates that the vast majority of librarians and knowledge specialists who join the health sector remain within it thereafter. Some may extend their role, for example, undertaking responsibilities for technology-enhanced learning. Some pursue career progression through embracing the management of other services, for example, where the library service is based in an education centre. Others may move out of the service into more senior roles within research governance infrastructures, in innovation or quality improvement, for example.

In future, working closely alongside health informatics colleagues may open up new avenues for career progression.

While very few knowledge specialists currently pursue a pathway into senior management roles within health service organisations, it is certainly possible – enabled by applying portable skills to a broader portfolio, gaining wider experience in management and investing in developing leadership skills. Greater alignment to clinical and executive teams is likely to facilitate this path. Becoming a senior manager opens up the potential to model optimum use of evidence, knowledge management tools and knowledge services to inform decision-making. It also affords opportunities to optimise the positioning and impact of knowledge services from an executive level. The health knowledge services of the future can only benefit from the influence of such senior managers.

Conclusion

Luck is what happens when preparation meets opportunity.

(Seneca the Younger)

A bright future lies ahead for healthcare knowledge services. Yet, this is not predetermined – it lies in our hands.

To quote Bill Gates:

We always overestimate the change that will occur in the next two years and underestimate the change that will occur in the next ten. Don't let yourself be lulled into inaction.

(Gates and Hemingway, 2000, 37)

Whatever scenarios unfold, the way forward is to prepare now.

As the Topol Review concluded:

There is now a window of opportunity in which to strengthen the infrastructure, upskill the workforce and catalyse the transformation. There is no time to waste.

(Topol, 2019, 82)

De facto it is through the continuous improvement of the services we offer today, through professional development and through preparation, that we can look to the future of healthcare knowledge services with confidence. Now is the time to press the case that health knowledge services are part of the solution to addressing the challenges facing healthcare systems across the world. Now is the time to redesign knowledge services and teams so that they are fit for the future. Now is the time to prepare to meet opportunity.

Do health knowledge services need to change? Absolutely. Will health knowledge services be vastly different in 15 years? Absolutely. Are knowledge specialists able to influence the route of travel? Absolutely. The issue is not whether health knowledge services will change but, rather, whether health knowledge specialists will change them sufficiently radically and sufficiently fast.

Be lucky.

References

Berwick, D. (2013) *Letter to the Clinicians, Managers and All Staff of the NHS.* https://assets.publishing.service.gov.uk/government/uploads/system/uploads/attachment_data/file/226709/berwick_letter_to_NHS.PDF.

Blaizot, A., Veettil, S. K. and Saidoung, P., Moreno-Garcia, C. F., Wiratunga, N., Aceves-Martins, M., Lai, N. M. and Chaiyakunapruk, N. (2022) Using Artificial Intelligence Methods for Systematic Review in Health Sciences: A Systematic Review, *Research Synthesis Methods*, **13** (3), 353–62. https://onlinelibrary.wiley.com/doi/abs/10.1002/jrsm.1553.

Braithwaite, J., Glasziou, P. and Westbrook, J. (2020) The Three Numbers You Need to Know About Healthcare: the 60-30-10 Challenge, *BMC Medicine*, **18**, 102. https://doi.org/10.1186/s12916-020-01563-4.

Brassey J., Price, C., Edwards, J., Zlabinger, M., Bampoulidis, A. and Hanbury, A. (2021) Developing a Fully Automated Evidence Synthesis Tool for Identifying, Assessing and Collating the Evidence, *BMJ Evidence-Based Medicine*, **26** (1), 24–7. https://ebm.bmj.com/content/26/1/24.

Brettle, A., Maden, M. and Payne, C. (2016) The Impact of Clinical Librarian Services on Patients and Health Care Organisations, *Health Information and Libraries Journal*, **33** (2), 100–20. https://onlinelibrary.wiley.com/doi/full/10.1111/hir.12136.

Bronsoler, A., Doyle, J. and Van Reenen, J., (2020) *The Impact of New Technology on the Healthcare Workforce*. https://workofthefuture.mit.edu/wp-content/uploads/2020/10/2020-Research-Brief-Bronsoler-Doyle-VanReenen.pdf.

Carlyle, R. (2022) Health and Digital Literacy: Addressing Inequalities, *Information Professional*, April/May, 33.

Carlyle, R., Crozier, J., Farrar, A., Hughes, S., James, S. and Thain, A. (2023) *Health Literacy: You Can Make a Difference*. Elearning for Healthcare. www.e-lfh.org.uk/programmes/healthliteracy.

Chartered Institute of the Library and Information Profession (CILIP) (2021) *The Professional Knowledge and Skills Base: Introduction and Overview, Developing Skills for Success*. https://cdn.ymaws.com/www.cilip.org.uk/resource/resmgr/cilip/membership/benefits/pksb/pksb_intro_overview_v5.pdf.

Cox, A. M. (2021) *The Impact of AI, Machine Learning, Automation and Robotics on the Information Profession. A Report for CILIP*. www.cilip.org.uk/general/custom.asp?page=researchreport.

Daugherty, P. R. and Wilson, H. J. (2018) *Human + Machine: Reimagining Work in the Age of AI*, Harvard Business Review Press.

Davenport, T. (1997) Known Evils, Common Pitfalls of Knowledge Management, *CIO Magazine*, June 15. http://web.archive.org/web/20061206151002/http:/www.cio.com:80/archive/061597/think.html.

Densen, P. (2011) Challenges and Opportunities Facing Medical Education, *Transactions of the American Clinical and Climatological Association*, **122**, 48–58. www.ncbi.nlm.nih.gov/pmc/articles/PMC3116346.

Department of Health and Social Care (2021) *Harnessing Technology for the Long-Term Sustainability of the UK's Healthcare System: Report.* www.gov.uk/government/publications/harnessing-technology-for-the-long-term-sustainability-of-the-uks-healthcare-system.

Economics by Design (2020) *NHS Funded Library and Knowledge Services in England – Value Proposition: The Gift of Time.* www.hee.nhs.uk/our-work/library-knowledge-services/value-proposition-gift-time.

Foley, T., Horwitz, L. and Zahran, R. (2021) *Realising the Potential of Learning Health Systems*, The Learning Healthcare Project. https://learninghealthcareproject.org/wp-content/uploads/2021/05/LHS2021report.pdf.

Gates, B. and Hemingway, C. (2000) *Business @ the Speed of Thought: Succeeding in the Digital Economy*, Warner Books.

General Medical Council (GMC) (2023) *Domain 1: Knowledge Skills and Performance.* www.gmc-uk.org/ethical-guidance/ethical-guidance-for-doctors/good-medical-practice/domain-1—-knowledge-skills-and-performance.

Gibson, M. (2015) *The Half Life of a Learned Skill is 5 years – Toward a New Culture of Learning.* www.whychangeselling.com/inbound-marketing-messaging-sales-performance-blog/bid/113040/the-half-life-of-a-learned-skill-is-5-years-toward-a-new-culture-of-learning.

Gilroy, D. (2021) New CILIP Professional Knowledge and Skills Base. *Blog. Health Education England Knowledge and Library Services*, 17 May. https://library.hee.nhs.uk/about/blogs/new-cilip-professional-knowledge-and-skills-base.

Glass, P. and Perkovic, V. (2021) *Affordability and Efficiency is the Future of Healthcare.* www.linkedin.com/pulse/affordability-efficiency-future-healthcare-parisa-glass.

Health Education England (2015) *Knowledge for Healthcare: A Development Framework (2015–2020).* www.hee.nhs.uk/sites/default/files/documents/Knowledge_for_healthcare_a_development_framework_2014.pdf.

Health Education England (2021a) *Knowledge for Healthcare: Mobilising Evidence; Sharing Knowledge; Improving Outcomes. A Strategic Framework for NHS Knowledge and Library Services 2021–2026.* www.hee.nhs.uk/our-work/knowledge-for-healthcare.

Health Education England (2021b) *KLS Statistical Return for NHS KLS Activity in England, 2020–21.* Unpublished.

Health Education England (2021c) *Artificial Intelligence in Specialist Search and Knowledge Management.*
https://library.hee.nhs.uk/resources/emerging-technologies/artificial-intelligence-in-specialist-search-and-knowledge-management.

Health Policy Partnership (2021) *Under Threat: Healthcare in Conflict Zones.*
www.healthpolicypartnership.com/under-threat-healthcare-in-conflict-zones.

Hutchinson, A., Slawson, D., Shaughnessy, A. and Underhill, J. (2012) *Information Mastery: Decision-Making and Dealing with Information Overload.* Supplementary web chapter in Mehay, R. (ed.), *The Essential Handbook for GP Training & Education*, Routledge.
www.essentialgptrainingbook.com/wp-content/online-resources/05%20information%20mastery.pdf.

International Federation of Library Associations (IFLA) (2012) *IFLA Code of Ethics for Librarians and other Information Workers (Full Version).* Approved by the IFLA Governing Board, August 2012.
https://repository.ifla.org/bitstream/123456789/1850/1/IFLA%20Code%20of%20Ethics%20for%20Librarians%20and%20Other%20Information%20Workers%20%28Long%20Version%29.pdf.

International Federation of Library Associations (IFLA) (2020) *Library Return on Investment: Reviewing the Evidence From the Last 10 years.*
https://cdn.ifla.org/wp-content/uploads/files/assets/hq/library_roi.pdf.

International Monetary Fund (IMF) (2022) *Patterns and Drivers of Health Spending Efficiency*, IMF Working Papers.
www.imf.org/en/Publications/WP/Issues/2022/03/04/Patterns-and-Drivers-of-Health-Spending-Efficiency-513694.

Ipsos MORI (2021a) *Ipsos MORI Veracity Index 2021 Trust in Professions Survey.* www.johnsmithcentre.com/research/ipsos-mori-veracity-index-2021-trust-in-professions-survey.

Ipsos MORI (2021b) *Ipsos Veracity Index: Trust in the Police Drops for the Second Year in a Row.* www.ipsos.com/en-uk/ipsos-mori-veracity-index-trust-police-drops-second-year-row.

Kearney (2020) *The Future of Work: Four Trends That Will Change Healthcare.* www.kearney.com/global-strategic-partnerships/world-economic-forum/article/-/insights/the-future-of-work-four-trends-that-will-change-healthcare.

McDonald, G. (2018) Advocating for Corporate Information Services, *CILIP News*, 10 July. www.cilip.org.uk/news/news.asp?id=434967.

McKinsey and Company (2021) *Defining the Skills Citizens Will Need in the Future World of Work*. www.mckinsey.com/industries/public-and-social-sector/our-insights/defining-the-skills-citizens-will-need-in-the-future-world-of-work.

McNally, R. (2021) *Clinical Librarians – A Personal View*, LKS North Blog, 19 January. www.lksnorth.nhs.uk/blog/posts/clinical-librarians-a-personal-view.

Maggio, L. A. and Artino, A. R. (2018) Staying Up To Date and Managing Information Overload, *Journal of Graduate Medical Education*, **10** (5), 597–8. www.ncbi.nlm.nih.gov/pmc/articles/PMC6194894.

Markoff, J. (2015) Planes Without Pilots, *New York Times*, 6 April, D1(L). www.nytimes.com/2015/04/07/science/planes-without-pilots.html.

New Zealand Institute of Economic Research (NZIER) (2016) *Digital Nation: New Zealand From a Tech Sector to Digital Nation*, NZIER, April. https://think-asia.org/bitstream/handle/11540/9216/digital_nation_nz.pdf?sequence=1. www.nzier.org.nz/hubfs/Public%20Publications/Client%20reports/digital_nation_nz.pdf.

NHS England (2019) *The NHS Long Term Plan*. www.longtermplan.nhs.uk/wp-content/uploads/2019/08/nhs-long-term-plan-version-1.2.pdf.

NHS Library and Knowledge Services in England (2020) *Recommendations to improve the staff ratio for the number of qualified library and knowledge specialists per member of NHS workforce*. www.hee.nhs.uk/sites/default/files/documents/HEE%20LKS%20Staff%20Ratio%20Policy%20January%202020.pdf

Nursing and Midwifery Council (NMC) (2018) *The Code: Professional Standards of Practice and Behaviour for Nurses, Midwives and Nursing Associates*. www.nmc.org.uk/globalassets/sitedocuments/nmc-publications/nmc-code.pdf.

O'Brien, N., Van Dael, J., Clarke, J., Gardner, C., O'Shaughnessy, J., Darzi, A. and Ghafur, S. (n.d.) *Addressing Racial and Ethnic Inequities in Datadriven Health Technologies*, Institute of Global Health Innovation, Imperial College London. https://spiral.imperial.ac.uk/bitstream/10044/1/94902/2/Imperial_IGHI_AddressingRacialandEthnicInequities%20_Report.pdf.

Ou, K., Felicia, P. and Kane, D. (2013) Using Simulations and Game-Based Learning for Information Skills Training, *Qualitative and Quantitative Methods in Libraries*, 2, 107–18. www.qqml-journal.net/index.php/qqml/article/view/85/86.

PWC (2023) *Health Services.*
www.pwc.com/gx/en/industries/healthcare/emerging-trends-pwc-healthcare/depleting-resources.html.

Sabey, A. and Biddle, M. (2021) Building Capacity Among Health Care Librarians to Teach Evidence-Based Practice – An Evaluation, *Journal of the Medical Library Association,* **109** (3), 432–40.
www.ncbi.nlm.nih.gov/pmc/articles/PMC8485954/pdf/jmla-109-3-432.pdf.

Sadera, G. (2019) *The Librarian as Knowledge Mobiliser in Critical Care: Summary,* Wirral University Teaching Hospital NHS Foundation Trust.

Sbaffi, L., Walton, J., Blenkinsopp, J. and Walton, G. (2020) Information Overload in Emergency Medicine Physicians: A Multisite Case Study Exploring the Causes, Impact, and Solutions in Four North England National Health Service Trusts, *Journal of Medical Internet Research,* **22** (7), e19126. www.ncbi.nlm.nih.gov/pmc/articles/PMC7418008.

St George's University (2021) *What Is Global Health? The 6 Biggest Issues You Need to Know About.* www.sgu.edu/blog/medical/what-is-global-health.

Sutton, R. T., Pincock, D., Baumgart, D.C., Sadowski, D. C, Fedorak, R. N. and Kroeker, K. I. (2020) An Overview of Clinical Decision Support Systems: Benefits, Risks, and Strategies for Success, *npj Digital Medicine,* **3**, 17. https://doi.org/10.1038/s41746-020-0221-y.

Topol, E. (2018) *Preparing the Healthcare Workforce to Deliver the Digital Future. Interim Report June 2018 – A Call for Evidence.*
www.hee.nhs.uk/sites/default/files/documents/Topol%20Review%20interim%20report_0.pdf.

Topol, E. (2019) *The Topol Review: Preparing the Healthcare Workforce to Deliver the Digital Future.* https://topol.hee.nhs.uk/wp-content/uploads/HEE-Topol-Review-2019.pdf.

United Nations (UN) (2022) *Sustainable Development Goals – 3: Ensure Healthy Lives and Promote Well-Being for All at All Ages.*
https://sdgs.un.org/goals/goal3.

van der Gaag, M., Heijmans, M., Ballestar, M., Orrego, C., Guzman, E., Ninov, L. and Rademakers, J. (2022) Preferences Regarding Self-Management Intervention Outcomes of Dutch Chronically Ill Patients With Limited Health Literacy, *Frontiers in Public Health,* **10**.
www.frontiersin.org/articles/10.3389/fpubh.2022.842462/full.

Vasey, B., Nagendran, M. and Campbell, B. et al. (2022) Reporting Guideline for the Early Stage Clinical Evaluation of Decision Support Systems Driven by Artificial Intelligence: DECIDE-AI, *BMJ,* 377, e070904.
www.bmj.com/content/377/bmj-2022-070904.

Walker, P. (2018) *What is the Academic Health Sciences Library's Role in the Learning Health Care System?* National Library of Medicine. https://nlmdirector.nlm.nih.gov/2018/07/17/learning-health-care-system.

Wickramarachchi, C. (2021) An Interview with an Emergency Medicine Doctor, Dr Wickramarachchi, *BMJ Best Practice*, 26 October. www.facebook.com/BMJBestPractice/photos/a.326586147473216/247935 0542196755/?type=3.

World Economic Forum (WEF) (2017) *Skill, Re-skill and Re-skill Again. How to Keep up With the Future of Work.* www.weforum.org/agenda/2017/07/skill-reskill-prepare-for-future-of-work.

World Health Organization (WHO) (2020) *Global Strategy on Human Resources for Health: Workforce 2030.* www.who.int/publications/i/item/9789241511131.

World Health Organization (WHO) (2021) *Climate Change and Health.* www.who.int/news-room/fact-sheets/detail/climate-change-and-health.

World Health Organization (WHO) (2022) *Ageing and Health.* www.who.int/news-room/fact-sheets/detail/ageing-and-health.

World Health Organization (WHO) (2023) *Noncommunicable Diseases.* www.who.int/news-room/fact-sheets/detail/noncommunicable-diseases.

Yamada, T., Yoneoka, D., Hiraike, Y., Hino, K., Toyoshiba, H., Shishido, A., Noma, H, Shojima, N. and Yamauchi, T. (2020) Deep Neural Network for Reducing the Screening Workload in Systematic Reviews for Clinical Guidelines: Algorithm Validation Study, *Journal of Medical Internet Research*, **22** (12), e22422. www.jmir.org/2020/12/e22422/PDF.

Index